Diabetes

Diabetes

Diabetes
Epidemiology, Pathophysiology and Clinical Management

Dr Awanish Kumar and Dr Ashwini Kumar

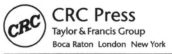

CRC Press is an imprint of the
Taylor & Francis Group, an **informa** business

Department of Biotechnology, National Institute of Technology, Raipur, Chhattisgarh, India
First edition published 2021

by CRC Press
6000 Broken Sound Parkway NW, Suite 300, Boca Raton, FL 33487-2742
and by CRC Press
2 Park Square, Milton Park, Abingdon, Oxon, OX14 4RN

ISBN: 9780367544591 (hbk)
ISBN: 9780367544577 (pbk)
ISBN: 9781003089391 (ebk)

Typeset in Frutiger
by Deanta Global Publishing Services, Chennai, India

Contents

Important Caveat

*This book is a compilation of various scientific facts and reports related to diabetes. These facts, or interpretation of any, **SHOULD NOT** be treated or inferred as medical advice. The authors highly discourage self-medication in any disease. Patients should always consult their doctor for their ailment.*

Preface

As the pathology of diabetes is ever increasing, it is hardly possible that anyone has not heard of it. People generally have experienced it either themselves, or with their family or close ones. Being metabolic in nature, diabetes has different facets. As we go on discussing and explaining every possible aspect of diabetes (as per our capacity and literature access) in this book, we thought it better to proceed with the global epidemiological scenario of the disease.

Chapter 1, therefore, deals with the global scenario of diabetes with updated figures and the basic classifications of diabetes. Moving ahead to **Chapter 2**, we explain how diabetes is an inflammatory disease. The underlying inflammatory mechanisms are discussed in a manner that is easy to understand. In **Chapter 3**, we explain the role and seriousness of insulin resistance which, we believe, remains largely neglected in various geographical locations. Establishing and explaining basic mechanisms leading to diabetes, we have included in **Chapter 4** how diabetes results in further comorbidities that at times become critical if the disease is not timely diagnosed and properly controlled. The diagnosis of any disease is the first consideration while the treatment follows thereafter. Thus, **Chapter 5** deals with various biomarkers that are useful in the diagnosis of diabetes. As mentioned, treatment follows diagnosis, and the therapeutic regimen is highly contingent on timely and accurate diagnosis. **Chapter 6**, therefore, deals with various drugs available for the war against diabetes. The chapter also includes various experimental drugs that are at different stages of development. **Chapter 7** deals with the various treatment modalities and protocols, including surgical procedures for extreme cases. Since diabetes is a multi-factorial pathology, proper combination of the drugs is crucial and depends upon the fine sense of judgement of the medical practitioner. Because of its metabolic nature, the treatment of diabetes does not completely depend upon the drugs. Initial management includes dietary and lifestyle modifications that are included in **Chapter 8**.

The authors hope and believe that the contents of this book can benefit a range of readers, from undergraduate science students to full-time researchers. Science opens up a new avenue every day. Therefore, we do not claim that we have covered all aspects of diabetes, but we can assure the reader that we have tried to create the best-possible content with up-to-date information within our capacity.

To finish, we would like to strongly emphasise the following: ***This book shall not be in any case treated as medical advice. Patients and caregivers are strongly discouraged from any kind of self-medication, while they are encouraged to consult their medical practitioner and dietician for proper advice***.

Wishing all the readers a great read.

Thanking you.

Awanish Kumar, PhD

Ashwini Kumar, PhD

Acknowledgements

It took us months to proceed with available literatures, evidence and other possible sources related to the contents of the chapters in our book. We are sure the readers will agree with us in stating that writing a book is a labour-intensive task which is performed with utmost care and precaution. In our process of writing this book, we acknowledge the kind support from the Department of Biotechnology, National Institute of Technology Raipur (Chhattisgarh), India.

Authors

Dr Awanish Kumar is an Assistant Professor in the Department of Biotechnology, National Institute of Technology, Raipur, India. He has more than 10 years of post-PhD research experience in the area of drug discovery and health care. He obtained his doctorate degree in 2009 from the Central Drug Research Institute (CDRI), Lucknow & Jawaharlal Nehru University (JNU), New Delhi, India and has undertaken post-doctoral study at McGill University, Montreal, Quebec, Canada. Dr Kumar has worked in various national and international organisations in different academic/research capacities. He has published more than 100 peer-reviewed research papers in SCI journals and he is the author of several books and chapters. Currently, he is working within various national institutional committees, scientific societies, advisory panels as well as actively contributing to academia and research. Dr Kumar has received numerous awards and accolades for his accomplishments. He is a member of many international professional research societies and is a reviewer/editorial board member of reputed and refereed journals.

Dr Ashwini Kumar obtained his MTech (Biotechnology) from the Department of Biotechnology & Medical Engineering, National Institute of Technology Rourkela (Odisha), India. His Master's research was focused on obesity, checking the effect of flavonoids on the lipid accumulation in adipocytes. He obtained his doctorate degree under the supervision of Dr Awanish Kumar at the Department of Biotechnology, National Institute of Technology Raipur (Chhattisgarh), India. The broad area of his doctoral research was the formulation of mucoadhesive drug delivery systems. His interest lies in biomaterials and metabolic diseases. He has 14 journal publications and seven book chapters to his credit. Currently, he is working as a Research Associate in the Department of Biochemical Engineering and Biotechnology, Indian Institute of Technology Delhi, India.

Abbreviations

3T3-L1:	3-day transfer, inoculum 3×10^5 cells; it is a mouse fibroblast cell line
A1MG:	Alpha-1 microglobulin
ACG:	American College of Gastroenterology
ACOG:	American College of Obstetricians and Gynecologists
AdipoR:	Adiponectin receptor
ADA:	American Diabetes Association
ADH:	Anti-diuretic hormone
AgRP:	Agouti-related peptide
AGE:	Advanced glycation end-products
AGI:	Alpha-glucosidase inhibitor
AHA:	American Heart Association
AIDS:	Acquired immunodeficiency syndrome
ALT:	Alanine transaminase
AMPK:	AMP-activated protein kinase
ApoA2:	Apo-lipoprotein A2
AQP2:	Aquaporin 2
AR:	Aldolase reductase
ARB:	Angiotensin receptor blockers
AVP:	Arginine vasopressin
BMI:	Body mass index
BNP:	Brain natriuretic peptide
CAD:	Coronary artery disease
CCR-2:	CC-chemokine receptor 2
CDC:	Center for Disease Control and Prevention, United States
C/EBP:	CAAT/enhancer binding protein
COPD:	Chronic obstructive pulmonary disorder
COX:	Cyclooxygenase
CRP:	C-reactive protein
CSII:	Continuous subcutaneous insulin infusion
CT:	Computed tomography

CVD:	Cardiovascular disorders
CysC:	Serum cystatin C
DC:	Dendritic cells
DCCT:	Diabetes Control and Complications Trial
DFI:	Diabetic foot infection
DI:	Diabetes insipidus
DKA:	Diabetes ketoacidosis
DLCO:	Diffusing capacity for carbon monoxide
DN:	Diabetic nephropathy
DPN:	Diabetic peripheral neuropathy
DPP:	Diabetes Prevention Program
DPP-4:	Dipeptide peptidase
DPPOS:	Diabetes Prevention Program Outcomes Study
DR:	Diabetic retinopathy
DSP:	Distal symmetric polyneuropathy
ECM:	Extracellular matrix
eGFR:	Estimated glomerular filtration rate
eNOS:	Endothelial nitric oxide synthase
ER:	Endoplasmic reticulum
ESRD:	End-stage renal disease
FDA:	Food and Drug Administration
FEV1:	Force expiratory volume in 1 second
FFA:	Free fatty acid
FGF:	Fibroblast growth factor
FMD:	Fast-mimicking diet
FPG:	Fasting plasma glucose
FVC:	Forced vital capacity
GAD:	Glutamic acid decarboxylase
GDM:	Gestational diabetes mellitus
GDP:	Gross domestic product
GFR:	Glomerular filtration rate
GI:	Glycaemic index
GK:	Glucokinase

GLP-1:	Glucagon-like peptide-1
GLUT:	Glucose transporter
GSIS:	Glucose-stimulated insulin secretion
HbA1c:	Glycosylated haemoglobin
HCC:	Hepatocellular carcinoma
HDL:	High-density lipoprotein
HFCS:	High-fructose corn syrup
HFD:	High-fat diet
HIV:	Human immunodeficiency virus
HLA:	Human leukocyte antigen
HMGB1:	High mobility group B1
HNF:	Hepatocyte nuclear factor
HSP:	Heat shock protein
HTN:	Hypertension
iNOS:	Inducible nitric oxide synthase
IAA:	Insulin autoantibodies
IADPSG:	International Association of the Diabetes and Pregnancy Study Groups
IAPP:	Islet amyloid polypeptide
ICA:	Islet cell antibodies
IDF:	International Diabetes Federation
IFG:	Impaired fasting glucose
IGT:	Impaired glucose tolerance
IL:	Interleukin
IR:	Insulin receptor
IRS:	Insulin receptor substrate
ISGU:	Insulin-stimulated glucose uptake
JDRF:	Juvenile Diabetes Research Foundation
JNK:	Janus kinase
kDa:	Kilodalton
KO:	Knock-out
LDL:	Low-density lipoprotein
LVH:	Left ventricular hypertrophy
MCP-1:	Monocyte chemoattractant protein-1

MDR: Multi-drug resistance

MDRF: Madras Diabetes Research Foundation

ME: Macular oedema

MMP: Matrix metalloproteinase

MODY: Maturity onset diabetes of the young

mRNA: Messenger ribonucleic acid

MRSA: Methicillin-resistant Staphylococcus aureus

MS: Metabolic syndrome

mTOR: Mammalian target of rapamycin

MUFA: Mono-unsaturated fatty acids

NADPH: Nicotinamide diadenosine phosphate

NAFLD: Non-alcoholic fatty liver disease

NASH: Non-alcoholic steatohepatitis

NEFA: Non-esterified fatty acids

NF-κB: Nuclear factor kappa beta

NGAL: Neutrophil gelatinase-associated lipocalin

NGSP: National Glycohemoglobin Standardization Program

NPH: Neutral protamine hagderon

NPY: Neuropeptide Y

NO: Nitric oxide

OGTT: Oral glucose tolerance test

PAI-1:   Plasminogen activator inhibitor-1

PAMP: Pathogen-associated molecular pattern

PARP: Poly ADP-ribose polymerase

PCOS: Polycystic ovary syndrome

PG: Plasma glucose

PI-3K: Phosphoinositide-3 kinase

PKB: Protein kinase B

PKC: Protein kinase C

PLA2:   Phospholipase A2

PLC: Phospholipase C

PPAR: Peroxisome proliferator-activated receptor

PPG: Post-prandial glucose

PTP:	Protein tyrosine phosphatase
PUFA:	Poly-unsaturated fatty acids
RAGE:	Receptor for AGE
RBP-4:	Retinol binding protein-4
RDS:	Respiratory distress syndrome
ROS:	Reactive oxygen species
RPG:	Random plasma glucose
SAA:	Serum amyloid A
SGLT-1/2:	Sodium glucose co-transporter-1/2
SNP:	Single nucleotide polymorphism
STAT:	Signal transduction and activator of transcription
SUR1:	Sulphonylurea receptor-1
SOCS3:	Suppressor of cytokine signalling 3
TACE:	TNF-alpha converting enzyme
T1DM:	Type 1 diabetes mellitus
T2DM:	Type 2 diabetes mellitus
TB:	Tuberculosis
TG:	Triglyceride or triacylglycerol
TLR:	Toll-like receptor
TNF:	Tumour necrosis factor
TTN:	Transient tachypnoea of the newborn
TZD:	Thiazolidinediones
USD:	US dollars
UTI:	Urinary tract infection
TZD:	Thiazolidinedione
VEGF:	Vascular endothelial growth factor
VGLUT1:	Vesicular glutamate transporter 1
VLDL:	Very low density lipoprotein
WHO:	World Health Organization

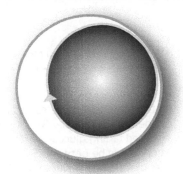

1 Diabetes Epidemiology – 1980 and Beyond

FACE-TO-FACE WITH THE GLOBAL DIABETES EPIDEMIOLOGY

In a global report on diabetes published by the World Health Organization (WHO) in 2016, almost 422 million people had diabetes in 2014 as compared to a figure of 108 million in 1980. Considering the adult population, global prevalence has almost doubled from 4.7% in 1980 to 8.5% in 2012. And the statistics don't stop there: 3.7 million deaths were recorded due to diabetes in 2012. Out of this number, almost 43% of deaths recorded were of people below 70 years of age. Aside from the health issues, diabetes has a large-scale global economic impact too. This includes the direct medical cost towards treatment, impact on professional work and premature mortality. The data presented by the WHO for the direct medical costs globally was approximately 827 billion USD. Sudden loss to life due to persistent diabetes poses a significant challenge to the family members of the deceased. Diabetes is also an indirect burden on national gross domestic product (GDP). In data presented by the WHO, it was estimated that worldwide GDP losses from 2011 to 2030 due to diabetes will be around 1.7 trillion USD [1]. In another estimate by the International Diabetes Federation (IDF), there will be around 642 million people in the world suffering from diabetes by 2040. Another report from the IDF, which is slightly contrasting, but points towards a bigger threat, says that there were approximately 3.96 million deaths due to diabetes (in the age group 20–79 years) in the year 2010, and this was expected to reach 5 million in 2015. Globally, around 45.8% of the total adult population suffering from diabetes goes undiagnosed, and therefore, these people are at greater risk of developing diabetes-related complications. Despite the large amount of undiagnosed cases of diabetes, the global economic burden is immense. It is estimated by the IDF that almost 673 billion USD (12% of global health expenditure) was spent on the treatment of diabetes and related comorbidities. In a relative estimate, the number of people with diabetes quadrupled from 1980 to 2014. It is also predicted that between 2010 and 2030, there will be an increase of 22% in the diabetic population in developed nations, while the figure soars to 69% in developing nations. The majority of this figure relates to type 2 diabetes mellitus (T2DM), which accounts for almost 90% of diagnosed diabetes cases; type 1 diabetes mellitus (T1DM), which is an autoimmune condition, accounts for the rest. Among specific nations, it has been shown that China and India are the diabetic (T2DM) epicentres of the world [2]. A large-scale population-based study in China suggested that it had a diagnosed diabetic population of almost 114 million and a pre-diabetic population of 494 million in 2010; while India had a diagnosed diabetic population of 62 million and a pre-diabetic population of 77 million in 2010. Among all this data, it is very important to mention that this population is the 'diagnosed' portion while many more cases are left undiagnosed. The criteria suggested and accepted globally for these diabetes and pre-diabetes ranges are impaired glucose tolerance defined as a figure of 7.8–11 mmol/L taken from a 2-hour oral glucose tolerance test, and impaired fasting glucose or fasting plasma glucose (FPG) of 5.6–6.9 mmol/L. The HbA1c value should be between 5.7–6.4% [2, 3]. Another report published in 2014 predicted that there would be around 592 million people with diabetes by 2015. The undiagnosed population could be yet more, as most of the people affected by diabetes are from low- and middle-income countries [4].

It is worth mentioning that this global burden of diabetes is highly attributed to lifestyle and environmental factors. Between the two broad types of diabetes, T2DM results either from prolonged insulin resistance, inability of insulin to act on the target tissues, decreased insulin production or sometimes a combination of these. The feedback loop between insulin production and insulin action gets disturbed, resulting in prolonged and persistent hyperglycaemia. Prolonged insulin resistance also results in increased hepatic glucose production. It has been reported that the incidence of diabetes in developed countries is highly attributed to the ever-increasing rate of obesity. On a global scale, the prevalence of obesity (which is defined as a BMI $\geq$30 kg/m^2) increased from 3.2% in 1975 to 10.8% in 2014 in men and from 6.4% to 14.9% in women. With this trend, it is predicted that the global incidence of obesity will reach 18% in men and more than 21% in women by 2025. Excess adiposity, either central or whole, is one of the greatest risk factors for T2DM. Extensive clinical trials and observations have suggested that lifestyle modifications can decrease the incidence of diabetes by almost 58%, which is much better than pharmacological interventions. Dietary patterns also suggested that high-quality fat and carbohydrates are much more effective in controlling diabetes and related problems than low-quality fat and carbohydrates [2]. A report on dietary factors suggests that consumption of processed red meat and sugar-sweetened beverages increases the incidence of T2DM while eating fruits and vegetables and whole grains reduces the chance [5].

One of the worst fears regarding diabetes is the high prevalence of undiagnosed diabetes. In a recent report from 2014 specifically on undiagnosed diabetes, it was estimated that about 45.8% of diabetes cases in adults globally is undiagnosed diabetes or newly diagnosed diabetes; almost 84% of these cases are in low- and middle-income nations. This is because the asymptomatic phase of T2DM can sustain for years while slowly negatively affecting the organs with complications such as cardiomyopathy, nephropathy, neuropathy and retinopathy, to name but a few. The rate of complications in undiagnosed diabetes cases is much higher than those in normoglycaemic people [6]. If we work with plain numbers, for example, this all amounts to approximately 23 million US citizens with 'diagnosed' diabetes, 7.2 million with undiagnosed diabetes, 1.5 million new diabetes cases every year and 84.1 million with pre-diabetes in 2015. In an estimated figure, the direct and indirect economic burden on the US economy due to diabetes was estimated to be 245 billion USD [7].

Talking about the science of the diabetes epidemic, diabetes is largely associated with genetic predisposition, environmental effects, developmental effects and lifestyle changes. On the one hand, where T1DM is an established autoimmune condition whereby the beta-islets are self-destructed by the body's immune system leading to insulin deficiency, T2DM is supposed to have a variety of causative factors. T2DM is also considered to be hereditary. On the specific genetic front, the monogenic form of diabetes, also known as maturity onset diabetes of the young (MODY), is considered to be caused by a specific genetic mutation. MODY, as per the definition, is diagnosed at adolescence or early adulthood [8]. MODY is autosomal dominant inherited diabetes which is hereditary too. As per the classification based on genetic mutation, MODY is classified as the hepatocyte nuclear factor 1α (HNF-1α) mutation type, HNF-4α mutation type, glucokinase (GK) mutation type and HNF-1β mutation type. In the HNF-1α mutation type, there is decreased production of insulin; it is responsible for almost 70% of MODY cases. It is the most common MODY in European nations such as Germany, Italy, Spain, Sweden and Finland while also frequently seen in Asian nations such as Japan and China. Patients with this mutation gradually present β-cell dysfunction resulting in hyperglycaemia. Owing to its progressive nature, the patient may, in the long term, develop microvascular and macrovascular diabetes-related complications. Patients with this type of MODY are extremely sensitive to sulphonylurea-related hypoglycaemia. Though they are initially treated with sulphonylurea, they might require insulin therapy over time. GK mutation is another very common type of MODY which presents by impaired glucose sensing mechanism by the pancreas. This disease displays mild non-progressive hyperglycaemia that may not be symptomatic. Most of the GK-mutation-type MODY patients maintain an HbA1c level below 8% and the patients usually do not develop any diabetes-related complications. The HNF-4α mutation type MODY is rare compared to the first two forms discussed above, and presents only in 2–5% of MODY cases. The patients also present gradual β-cell dysfunction and they are diagnosed with diabetes usually before the age of 25. The patients with this form of MODY may also develop reduced serum HDL cholesterol due to decreased ApoA2 transcription. A foetus with this mutation tends to have a higher birth weight, along with macrosomia. There are also cases of transient neonatal hypoglycaemia in children before the actual diagnosis of diabetes. The patients are prone to developing diabetes-related complications and might require gradual insulin therapy [9–11]. One of the major problems associated with MODY is the diagnostic delay. Currently, the diagnosis is made on the basis of genetic testing or gene sequencing that is widely available in developed countries. But the delay from the patients' side in approaching their doctor or the delay in detecting the strong family history of diabetes results in an average 13-year delay in MODY diagnosis in the UK. It is suggested that general practitioners, if there are doubts around MODY, should refer the patient to a local centre specialising in diabetes or genetic testing to get the condition confirmed. The patients should undergo genetic counselling and the immediate family members should also be advised to get tested for the condition. The second most common cause of delay is that most cases of MODY are often misdiagnosed as T1DM or T2DM. The diagnosis must consider the endogenous production of C-peptide and ketoacidosis (in the case of T1DM) and insulin resistance and β-cell function (in the case of T2DM) within 3–5 years of initial diagnosis [12]. Thus, MODY, in its true form, is genetic in nature and can easily turn out to be heritable.

According to a very recent meta-analysis by the IDF, high- and middle-income countries had a higher prevalence of diabetes as compared to lower-income countries, while almost 75% of people with diabetes live in lower- or middle-income countries. It was also reported that over 50% of the adult population with diabetes goes undiagnosed in South-East Asia and the Western Pacific region. Global diabetes health expenditure was reported to be around 673 billion USD in 2015, and it is projected to be around 802 billion USD in 2040. The severity of diabetes-related deaths can be seen from the fact that the total number of mortalities due to diabetes (approximately 5 million in 2015) was more than the combined mortality figure for HIV/AIDS, tuberculosis and malaria. Therefore, explaining diabetes epidemiology in short, it is reported that diabetes is perhaps one of the fastest-growing diseases globally that affects both rural and urban populations. The only problematic difference is that due to a lack of proper healthcare facilities in rural regions of developing and underdeveloped countries, a great portion of the population may remain undiagnosed which may result in diabetes-related complications that ultimately deteriorate the quality of life [13]. In the 'Standards of Medical Care in Diabetes – 2018' report by the American Diabetes Association (ADA), it was reported that the percentage of the diabetic population that have achieved the recommended target HbA1c, LDL and blood pressure level has decreased. The mean value of HbA1c in the United States has decreased from 7.6% (60 mmol/mol) between 1999 and 2002 to 7.2% (55 mmol/mol) between 2007 and 2010, as per the report by the National Health and Nutrition Examination Survey. Apart from that, late diagnosis (or even misdiagnosis) of diseases is a significant factor towards overall increase in health expenditure globally that might result in increased diabetes-related mortality too [13]. The problem of limited healthcare in rural regions as stated above could be brought under control by the system of telemedicine. Telemedicine is the application of telecommunication to make required basic healthcare accessible to remote geographical regions. Food insecurity is another major geographical problem which leads to people not getting the adequate amount of food and nutrition. Such a population might be largely dependent on a specific type of food such as those containing a high amount of starch or carbohydrates. It was also reported that the risk of T2DM has increased almost two-fold in populations with food insecurity. In such a population, there is a risk of both uncontrolled hyperglycaemia (due to high consumption of inexpensive carbohydrate and carbohydrate-rich processed foods, binge eating or financial problems) and sudden hypoglycaemia (due to inadequate carbohydrate consumption followed by taking sulphonylureas or insulin) [3]. Apart from the normal T1DM and T2DM, there is a third type of diabetes that is considered only in pregnancy and is referred to as gestational diabetes mellitus (GDM). It is generally defined as hyperglycaemia in women at 24–28 weeks of their pregnancy with a non-existence of any previous diabetes. It is also recommended that women with GDM be screened for diabetes 4–12 weeks postpartum using an oral glucose tolerance test (OGTT) and they must also be screened for diabetes every 3 years. The diagnosis of GDM is generally made by two different approaches. The first approach is a one-step process where an OGTT is performed with 75 grams of glucose after at least 8 hours of fasting in the morning at 1 hour and 2 hours. The second approach is a two-step process where a glucose load test is firstly performed in a non-fasting state with 50 grams of glucose at 1 hour. If the plasma glucose level is recorded ≥140 mg/dl, a 3-hour 100-gram glucose OGTT should be performed in a fasting state. However, the International Association of Diabetes and Pregnancy Study Groups (IADPSG) recommend the one-step strategy as the preferred approach [3].

As a general note and information to all readers, the diagnosis of diabetes, in general, as described by the ADA is as follows [3]:

1. A fasting plasma glucose (FPG) ≥126 mg/dl (7 mmol/L) after fasting of at least 8 hours
   OR
2. 2-hour plasma glucose ≥200 mg/dl (11.1 mmol/L) with a 75-gram oral glucose tolerance test
   OR
3. HbA1c ≥6.5% (48 mmol/mol)

Thus, we see that a lot of biological, environmental, genetic, financial and habitual factors are involved in the development of prolongation of both T1DM and T2DM. Whereas insulin remains the only therapeutic option for T1DM patients, T2DM patients have other orally available medication options that are considered for an initial therapeutic regimen.

Dietary factors serve largely in maintaining the recommended glycaemic level in diabetic subjects and thus diet control and lifestyle modification are highly recommended for patients with diabetes.

A rare type of diabetes, though not associated with hyperglycaemia, is diabetes insipidus (DI). It has been called 'diabetes' because of the central characteristic of excessive water loss through urination, which is also one of the cardinal signs of uncontrolled diabetes. The excessive loss of water through urination has been attributed to the peptide hormone vasopressin, also known as anti-diuretic hormone (ADH) or arginine vasopressin (AVP). The loss of function or loss of signalling to this hormone is the primary reason for DI. Largely, DI has been classified as central, nephrogenic, dipsogenic and gestational. Vasopressin or ADH, as the name suggests, control the fluid loss through urine. In central DI, there is damage to the hypothalamus or pituitary gland which results in a decrease or loss of ADH production and action. This results in loss of control in the amount of water lost through urine. Nephrogenic DI occurs when the kidneys fail to respond to the normal level of vasopressin; consequently there is excessive water loss. It can occur due to reasons such as chronic kidney disease, mutation in the vasopressin receptors in the kidneys, medications such as lithium, high blood calcium and low potassium in the blood. Since there is supposedly a feedback loop in vasopressin-water intake, dipsogenic DI occurs when there is damage to the thirst signalling located in the hypothalamus. As a result, a large intake of water suppresses vasopressin release which results in increased urine output. It is worth highlighting that gestational DI occurs relatively rarely. Major symptoms of DI include excessive thirst, fatigue and dry skin, while seizures and brain damage due to severe dehydration occur rarely [14]. The level of thirst could be severe enough to consume up to 20 litres of water per day. As a result of this huge water consumption, there is a rapid increase in the amount of urine. Thus, excessive water loss may result in hypovolaemia and electrolyte imbalance. The ADH maintains the water balance in normal individuals by acting on the vasopressin-2-receptor (V2R) upon detecting blood osmolarity and the arterial blood volume. ADH activates V2R present in the basolateral membrane of the principal cells in the renal collecting duct and distal convoluted tubule. This interaction activates protein kinase A (PKA) which results in phosphorylation of aquaporin 2 (AQP2) water channels in the intracellular vesicles. This activation is followed by the translocation of AQP2 vesicles into the cell membrane that exposes the AQP2. The collecting duct becomes water permeable due to AQP2 and concentrates the urine resulting in control of water loss [15].

The occurrence of DI is rare with a frequency of 1 in 25,000 cases. The genetic cause contributes to less than 10% of total cases. As per the frequency, central DI is the most common and can occur at any age. Since the hypothalamus is the site of expression and formation of vasopressin, while the pituitary aids in secretion of the hormone, any damage to the hypothalamus and pituitary could impair vasopressin production and secretion. It is reported that central DI manifestation generally occurs only after damage to 80% to 90% of vasopressin-associated neurons in the hypothalamus. Pituitary tumours, hypothalamic tumours and pituitary surgeries could also result in central DI. In the case of nephrogenic DI, the urine output could still be around 12L/day. Most nephrogenic DI cases are an X-linked mutation that results in mutated V2R resulting in loss of function. Only around 10% of cases occur due to a mutation in the AQP2 gene. Apart from the genetic cause, the lithium drug, foscarnet and clozapine cause drug-induced nephrogenic DI. In addition to the damage caused from the sensation of thirst, dipsogenic DI can also have a psychiatric impact, mostly due to obsessive compulsive disorders. Anti-cholinergic drugs administered in the psychiatric care of some patients might also result in the sensation of excessive thirst, thus resulting in increased water intake [15].

Thus, whereas T1DM, T2DM and gestational diabetes are associated with hyperglycaemia and related comorbidities, diabetes insipidus is concerned only with polydipsia and polyuria and related comorbidities.

REFERENCES

1. Global report on diabetes; WHO, 2016.
2. Zheng Y, Ley SH, Hu FB. Global aetiology and epidemiology of type 2 diabetes mellitus and its complications. *Nat Rev Endocrinol* 2018;14(2):88–98.
3. American Diabetes Association. Classification and diagnosis of diabetes: Standards of medical care in diabetes. *Diabetes Care* 2018;41(Suppl. 1):S13–S27.
4. Guariguata L, Whiting DR, Hambleton I, Beagley J, Linnenkamp U, Shaw JE. Global estimates of diabetes prevalence for 2013 and projections for 2035. *Diabetes Res Clin Pract* 2014;103(2):137–149.
5. Norouhi NG, Wareham NJ. Epidemiology of diabetes. *Medicine (Abingdon)* 2014;42(12):698–702.
6. Beagley J, Guariguata L, Weil C, Motala AA. Global estimates of undiagnosed diabetes in adults. *Diabetes Res Clin Pract* 2014;103(2):150–160.
7. Accessed at www.diabetes.org/diabetes-basics/statistics/; accessed on May 7, 2018.
8. Accessed at www.niddk.nih.gov/health-information/diabetes/overview/what-is-di abetes/monogenic-neonatal-mellitus-mody#3; accessed on May 9, 2018.
9. Accessed at www.diabetes.org.uk/diabetes-the-basics/other-types-of-diabetes/m ody; accessed on May 10, 2018.
10. Gardner DSL, Tai ES. Clinical features and treatment of maturity onset diabetes of the young (MODY). *Diabetes Metab Syndr Obes* 2012;5:101–108.
11. Nyunt O, Wu JY, McGown IN, Harris M, Huynh T, Leong GM et al. Investigating maturity onset diabetes of the young. *Clin Biochem Rev* 2009;30(2):67–74.
12. Thanabalasingham G, Owen KR. Diagnosis and management of maturity onset diabetes of the young (MODY). *BMJ* 2011;343:d6044.
13. Ogurtsova K, da Rocha Fernandes JD, Huang Y, Linnenkamp U, Guariguata L et al. IDF Diabetes Atlas: Global estimates for the prevalence of diabetes for 2015 and 2040. *Diabetes Res Clin Pract* 2017. doi: 10.1016/j.diabres.2017.03.024.
14. Accessed at www.niddk.nih.gov/health-information/kidney-disease/diabetes-insi pidus. Accessed on 10 May, 2019.
15. Kalra S, Zargar AH, Jain SM, Sethi B, Chowdhury S, Singh AK et al. Diabetes insipidus: The other diabetes. *Indian J Endocrinol Metab* 2016;20(1):9–21.

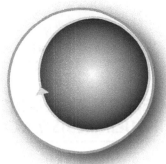

2 Diabetes and Inflammation

INTRODUCTION

Diabetes mellitus is generally classified into two broad categories, namely type 1 diabetes or T1DM and type 2 diabetes or T2DM. The first one is an autoimmune disorder where the pancreatic β-cells are self-destroyed, and this type accounts for approximately 5% of total diabetes incidences around the globe. The second type, i.e. T2DM, is the most prevalent and accounts for almost 95% of total diabetic subjects in the world. T2DM is very frequently related to obesity; more commonly than its genetic predisposition.

Inflammation is a state developed due to interplay among a lot of pro-inflammatory cytokines secreted and the cells involved, leading to patho-physiological immune activation. In other words, the secretion of pro-inflammatory cytokines is suggestive of inflammation. The association between inflammation and insulin resistance was first made about a century ago but the exact mechanism was not understood. Wilhelm Ebstein, in 1876, found that glycosuria disappeared in probable diabetic patients when salicylic acid was administered to them. In 1957, it was rediscovered that diabetic subjects with severe arthritis displayed obvious glycosuria, but the condition disappeared when they were treated with aspirin (salicylic acid), which was for the arthritic condition. Much later, it was found that the mechanism was dependent on the inhibition of nuclear factor-κB (NF-κB), a gene greatly involved in inflammation [1]. Obesity results in a state of chronic inflammation due to activation of the innate immune system resulting in high circulation of inflammatory cytokines such as tumour necrosis factor-α (TNF-α), interleukin-6 (IL-6), interleukin 1β (IL-1β) and many others. Macrophage infiltration in adipose tissue also results in increased TNF-α secretion from these macrophages. These cytokines have been shown to disrupt the anabolic insulin signalling, thus blocking insulin action. Resulting inflammation also leads to an increase in acute phase proteins such as C-reactive protein (CRP), plasminogen activator inhibitor-1 (PAI-1) and others. The adipose tissue has also been seen to be extensively inhabited by macrophages. It is seen that chronic high levels of pro-inflammatory cytokines make individuals more susceptible towards T2DM. People who are genetically predisposed towards T2DM have higher levels of pro-inflammatory cytokines as well. Administration of TNF-α or IL-6 in experimental rodents led to insulin resistance and eventual T2DM, while anti-TNF-α molecule resulted in improved insulin sensitivity and glucose homeostasis. It was also reported that expression of toll-like receptors (TLRs) is increased and binds with FFA and leads to obesity-induced insulin resistance [1, 2]. In the present chapter, the role of inflammatory cytokines as causative agents of insulin resistance and T2DM will be discussed so to be easily understood by anyone from undergraduate level and above.

GENERAL MECHANISM OF INFLAMMATION-INDUCED INSULIN RESISTANCE

Two decades ago, Hotamisligil et al. reported that inflammatory cytokine TNF-α, actively secreted from adipose tissue, is involved in inducing insulin resistance and affected glucose metabolism. TNF-α mRNA expression in adipocytes and TNF-α serum concentration were elevated considerably in obesity [3]. Adipose tissue was reported to be one of the sites of production of other important inflammatory cytokines such as IL-6, IL-1β, PAI-1, retinol binding protein-4 (RBP-4), serum amyloid A (SA-A) and many more. Pro-inflammatory cytokines TNF-α and IL-1β also activate the NF-κB and JNK, which are one of the most important transcription factors acting as an inflammation activator. NF-κB is also activated by TLR activation by free saturated fatty acids and, along with activated c-Jun N-terminal kinase (JNK), it phosphorylates serine/threonine residues of the insulin receptor substrate-1 (IRS-1) making it inactive. Ceramides, the precursor of sphingolipids, are also increased in obesity which activate NF-κB leading to inflammatory stress [1].

Another important mechanism reported is the endoplasmic reticulum (ER) stress in adipocytes and hepatocytes due to lipid accumulation, as seen in obesity. This ER stress results in the inactivation of IRS-1 by phosphorylating it at the serine/threonine residue. Monocyte chemoattractant protein-1 (MCP-1) is an important cytokine secreted by adipocytes which plays an important role in recruiting monocytes and dendritic cells (DCs), the most important immune cells involved in inflammation, at adipose tissue sites. Thus, it can be seen that almost all the pro-inflammatory cytokines and cells play a role in insulin resistance and gradual T2DM [2].

Macrophage Activation and Insulin Resistance in Obesity

Obesity is characterised by adipocyte hyperplasia resulting in their stress condition and increases the release of free fatty acids (FFA). Fatty acid dysregulation and endoplasmic reticulum (ER) stress, thus, are some of the main occurrences in obesity and these FFA are said to be the factor triggering the inflammatory macrophage activation. Saturated fatty acids (SFAs), but not unsaturated fatty acids (USFAs), are responsible for this classical inflammatory activation of macrophages in the adipose tissue region resulting in an inflammatory response. These SFAs are said to bind with toll-like receptor-4 (TLR4) resulting in macrophage activation in adipose tissue followed by increasing insulin resistance. CC-chemokine receptor 2 (CCR2) or monocyte chemoattractant protein-1 (MCP-1) is another important surface molecule on monocytes which trigger their trafficking into tissue, where they become macrophages and gain inflammatory activation. It has been shown in animal models that a lack of CCR2 results in failure of monocytes from getting recruited into adipose tissue [4]. It was also shown that classical macrophage activation resulted in activation of JNK and NF-κB, resulting in diminished insulin signalling [5]. In another ground-breaking study, it was shown that hyperglycaemia induces increased expression of TLR2 and TLR4 in circulating monocytes via the protein kinase C enzyme (PKC), further worsening the inflammatory response [6]. Since it is a well-known immunology fact that macrophages are one of the largest *in vivo* producers of pro-inflammatory cytokines, it is very obvious that a large outflow of such cytokines would result in insulin resistance as discussed later.

Uncontrolled hyperglycaemia is frequently associated with atherosclerosis. It has been observed that in the hyperglycaemic state, the expression of the monocyte receptor,

CD14, is increased on endothelial cells. These monocytes later become macrophages on phagocytosing circulating lipids. The expression of pro-inflammatory cytokines and chemokines is also elevated in monocytes in response to hyperglycaemia. Monocyte adhesion is also increased in the hyperglycaemic state. These activated monocytes, when converted to macrophages, start secreting TNF-α and IL-6, which is a potent atherogenic cytokine and may increase the cardiovascular risk by up to three times. In diabetic subjects, it was also found that TNF-α and IL-8 have positive correlation and show atherosclerotic synergism. IL-8 also recruits granulocytes and T-cells, increasing their cytotoxicity and thus inflammatory activity [7]. Table 2.1 lists some of the most common inflammatory factors and markers involved in T2DM.

Table 2.1 Inflammatory Factors and Markers Involved in T2DM

Factors/ Markers	Action Mediated
TNF-α	Increased secretion by macrophages infiltrating adipose tissue, Inhibits IR autophosphorylation, Inhibits IRS-1 phosphorylation, Elevated triglyceride and VLDL, Inhibition of GLUT-4 translocation in adipocytes and skeletal muscle cells, Downregulates the PPAR-γ and C/EBP-α expression, Induces PTP-1B activity which suppresses IRS-1 signalling.
Interleukins	IL-6 is increased in obesity and increases triglyceride and VLDL, Trigger the release of CRP, Increased risk of atherosclerosis, Interaction with IL-1β is responsible for actions of IL-6, Impaired insulin secretion due to increased Fas signalling and β-cell apoptosis, IL-1 antagonism results in improved peripheral insulin sensitivity, IL-13 attenuates insulin resistance, IL-17 destroys β-cells, IL-17 increase COX-2 and downregulates BCL-2.
CRP	Induced by IL-6, Positively related to endothelial dysfunction, Induces secretion of adipokines responsible for insulin resistance, High prevalence in diabetic women, IL-6 increases in central obesity, Higher risk of atherosclerosis, Activates β-cell apoptosis, Increased formation of foam cells.
TLRs	Induce innate immune response, AGEs activate TLR-2 and TLR-4, Increased formation of foam cells, Hyperglycaemia induces TLR expression on immune cells resulting in NF-κB activation, Increased oxidation of macromolecules due to elevated superoxide.
Macrophages	SFA activates the adipose tissue macrophages, Classical activation results in activation of JNK and NF-κB resulting in insulin resistance, Hyperglycaemia increases CD14 receptor expression on endothelial surface resulting in increased monocytes adhesion.
Others	Adipocytes, in obesity, secrete RBP-4, SAA and PAI-1, which are positively related to insulin resistance and related pathological consequences, Ceramides are increased in obesity which increases insulin resistance, Obesity increases ER stress in adipocytes and hepatocytes resulting in IRS-1 inactivation

ROLE OF PRO-INFLAMMATORY CYTOKINES IN DIABETES

Tumour Necrosis Factor – α

TNF-α is expressed as a 26-kDa membrane protein which gets cleaved by the TNF-α converting enzyme (TACE), releasing a 17-kDa fragment which is the main functional molecule. TNF-α is the primary pro-inflammatory cytokine released mainly by macrophages resulting from bacterial infection. But it is seen that macrophages which infiltrate adipose tissue also secrete TNF-α and in obesity this secretion increases by almost 2.5 times. It was also found that inhibition of TNF-α led to an improvement in insulin sensitivity. Body weight reduction also led to a decrease in total serum TNF-α leading to a reduction in insulin resistance [2]. TNF-α has also been shown to inhibit the insulin receptor (IR) autophosphorylation, phosphorylation of IRS-1 and activity of Akt disrupting the insulin signalling cascade. TNF-α administration in vivo also resulted in elevated serum triglyceride and very low-density lipoprotein (VLDL) due to increased hepatic lipogenesis. Another important effect of TNF-α on adipocytes and skeletal muscle cells is the inhibition of the GLUT-4 receptor, which is the primary receptor responsible for glucose intake in the cells [8, 9].

TNF receptor 2 (TNFR2) is occasionally shed from the membrane on binding of TNF-α, giving soluble TNF receptor 2 (sTNFR2). It has been seen that in diabetic subjects, this shedding increases and concentration of sTNFR2 is negatively correlated with insulin sensitivity [10]. In insulin-resistant individuals, the mRNA level of TNF-α in skeletal muscle cells was found to be higher than in control subjects. TNF-α administration is also shown to downregulate the expression of peroxisome proliferator activated receptor-γ (PPAR-γ) and CAAT/enhancer binding protein-α (C/EBP-α) which are transcription factors related to positive insulin sensitivity. This is also one of the important mechanisms of TNF-α induced insulin resistance. This is also supported by the fact that PPAR-γ agonists, thiazolidinedione (TZDs), suppress TNF-α expression owing to the improvement of the insulin sensitivity in diabetic individuals. TNF-α administration was also found to induce the protein tyrosine phosphatase-1B (PTP-1B) activity resulting in dephosphorylation of IRS-1 protein, thus inhibiting the downstream insulin signalling [11].

Interleukins

Interleukins are another very important pro-inflammatory cytokine released from a variety of cells such as macrophages, adipocytes, endothelial cells and epithelial cells. Some of the important interleukins involved and studied in inflammation mediated insulin resistance and T2DM are IL-6, IL-1β, IL-8. On the other hand, IL-13 has been found to attenuate insulin resistance and plays a positive role in insulin sensitivity.

Interleukin-6 (IL-6) secretion is increased in obesity and is involved in accelerated hepatic VLDL secretion and hypertriglyceridaemia. One of the most important acute phase proteins, CRP, which is released from the liver, is also triggered by IL-6. There have been many human studies suggesting a direct positive relation between IL-6 level and incident T2DM, which was shown to be independent of obesity. Various polymorphisms also exist in the IL-6 and Il-6 receptor (IL6R). The two most common single nucleotide polymorphisms (SNPs) in the promoter region of IL-6, rs1800795 (-174 G>C) and rs1800796 (-572 G>C), have been shown for their role in the predisposition to T2DM [2]. In a study more than a decade ago by Duncan et al., it was shown that the IL-6 level was strongly associated with glucose level and it is a good marker for the risk of T2DM and related atherosclerosis. It was also found in a few studies relating to IL-6 and HbA1c that the IL-6 level was elevated in people in whom HbA1c was greater than 6.5% [12]. Another important study about a decade ago reflects a clear, more exploratory relation between IL-6 and T2DM. The researchers showed that T2DM patients had significantly high levels of both IL-6 and IL-1β, where both are said to interact with each other, while an increase in IL-6 alone was not significantly associated with T2DM. This interaction of IL-6 and IL-1β increased the risk of T2DM by almost three times [13].

High blood glucose leads to elevated IL-1β production from pancreatic β-cells which results in impaired insulin secretion and finally the destruction of β-cells through increased Fas signalling, which is known as autocrine apoptosis. This β-cell apoptosis gradually leads to a decrease in β-cell mass leading to significantly reduced insulin secretion [14]. Pancreatic β-cells from T2DM patients had high levels of IL-1β as compared to non-diabetic patients. The application of the IL-1 receptor antagonist in diabetic rats reduced the secretion of pro-inflammatory cytokines from islets, improved insulin sensitivity and reduced the proinsulin/insulin ratio, finally decreasing hyperglycaemia. These animal models also exhibited fewer or reduced hepatic inflammatory markers. The IL-1 receptor antagonist also reduced the peripheral inflammation, thus improving peripheral insulin sensitivity [15]. The IL-8 level was also found to be directly related to diabetes. This elevation in IL-8 was found to be directly in consensus with high TNF-α but was not released by adipocytes, and thus has low concentration in obesity. It has recently been shown that the B-cell is activated in obesity due to TLR-2 activation resulting in elevated secretion of IL-8 [16].

IL-17 is a new class of interleukins which was shown to be actively involved in autoimmune diseases including T1DM, and also the non-autoimmune T2DM. IL-17, in co-ordination with Th17 immune cells (a new modified T-helper cell involved in autoimmune pathologies), has been very active in T1DM by directly influencing the destruction of pancreatic β-cells, since these cells have high expression of IL-17 receptors. Interferon-γ (IFN-γ), secreted by TH17 cells, is one of the major molecules destroying β-cells in T1DM. IL-17 has also been shown to upregulate COX-2 and downregulate the anti-apoptotic BCL-2 gene which are greatly responsible for β-cell dysfunction and damage. This IL-17 mediated immunity was shown to be present in people with recent as well as past T1DM [17]. In another study, it was reported that IL-17 is greatly produced by a new subset of NKT cells known as iNKT cells (invariant NKT cells) and highly involved in pathogenesis of T1DM. The study found an increment in these cells in the pancreas of T1DM patients. IL-17 and IFN-γ induce high iNOS expression in β-cells resulting in dysfunctional β-cells [18].

C – Reactive Protein (CRP)

CRP is a one of the most important hepatic acute phase proteins secreted and involved in inflammation. It is derived from the liver in response to IL-6. Thus, an increase in IL-6 in T2DM leads to elevated CRP. In a large human population study, it was found that IL-6 and the CRP level were elevated in diabetic subjects as compared to the normal controls. Elevated CRP has also been found to be positively associated with endothelial dysfunction. Increased IL-6 and CRP also stimulate the adipocytes to release further adipose-derived molecules responsible for insulin resistance. CRP level is also positively correlated with serum insulin, which is suggestive of a strong insulin resistance. In one study, it was concluded, interestingly, that CRP was a T2DM predictor in women but not in men. It was also shown that adipocytes from omental fat (central obesity) secreted two to three times higher IL-6 than those from the subcutaneous adipocytes. Between IL-6 and downstream protein CRP, the latter was found to be a better marker for future incidence of T2DM [19]. It has been noticed that obese subjects with elevated CRP have twice the risk of developing T2DM within 3–4 years. Higher CRP is also related to a higher risk of atherosclerosis [20]. CRP has also been shown to be a marker since it was found to be elevated in healthy subjects who developed T2DM later in life. It was estimated that one-third of total T2DM subjects have elevated CRP. CRP is also actively involved in decreasing insulin production by activating β-cell apoptosis by modulating cellular protein kinase B (PKB). Certain SNPs, such as rs3093059 and rs2794521, in the *CRP gene* were found to be positively correlated to the development of T2DM [21]. CRP has also been shown to increase the LDL uptake by macrophages converting them to pro-atherogenic foam cells. It was found that non-diabetic subjects with a family history of T2DM had higher circulating CRP than the age- and BMI-matched subjects from non-T2DM families [22].

Toll-Like Receptors

Toll-like receptors (TLRs) belong to a special class of surface molecules, found on immune cells, which recognise pathogen-associated molecular pattern (PAMP) and were originally found to be involved in inflammatory reaction against pathogenic attack. These TLRs, as a result, induce innate immune responses. These receptors are also activated by exogenous and endogenous non-microbial ligands, such as fatty acids, resulting in the release of cytokines. The two major TLRs involved in inflammatory response are TLR-2 and TLR-4. Some exogenous and endogenous ligands for these receptors are high mobility group B1 (HMGB1), necrotic cells, hyaluronic acid fragments, serum amyloid A (SAA) and advanced glycation end products (AGEs). These two TLRs are the most important among this family of receptors which play a very important inflammatory role in the development of atherosclerosis. Their expression is also seen to be increased dramatically in macrophages involved in the development of foam cells in atherosclerosis. TLR-2 and TLR-4 expression, their downstream signalling and inflammation are seen to be positively correlated with HbA1c levels in type 1 diabetic (T1DM) subjects [6, 23].

One recent study showed that high glucose concentration or hyperglycaemia results in significant increase in the expression of TLR-2 and TLR-4 in human monocytes cell lines and the monocytes isolated from diabetic subjects, resulting in NF-κB activation and eventual inflammatory response. TLR-2 and TLR-4 expression is also observed in a variety of other cells such as endothelial cells, coronary artery smooth muscle cells, adipocytes and pancreatic islets. It was also found experimentally that high glucose induced increased TLR-2 and TLR-4 expression persists for around 2–3 days before coming back to normal if hyperglycaemia is reduced to normal levels. It was also shown that hyperglycaemia leads to increased superoxide release from monocytes, which is a potent oxidising agent [6]. This increase in TLR expression is positively correlated with insulin resistance, N-carboxymethyllysine (N-CML), which is an important physiological

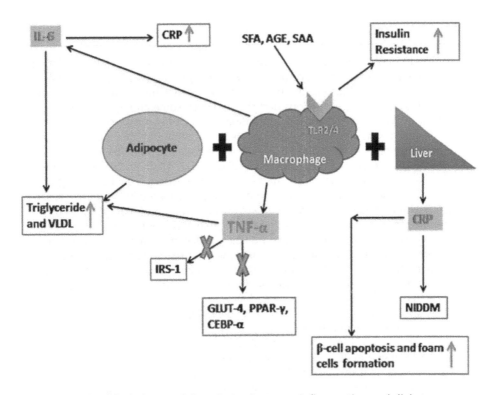

Figure 2.1 A simplified picture of the relation between inflammation and diabetes.

AGE and FFA. The concentration and number of ligands for these two TLRs, such as heat shock protein 60 (HSP 60), HSP 70 and HMGB1, are also increased and were consistent with hyperglycaemia. HMGB1 is a chromatin protein similar to histone which is released by immune cells, mostly monocytes, macrophages and dendritic cells. In a few reported studies, it was shown that certain drug classes such as thiazolidinediones (TZDs), statins and angiotensin receptor blockers (ARBs) decrease the TLR expression [24] (Figure 2.1).

CONCLUSIONS

Inflammation is a protective immune response of the body against a variety of foreign invasions. It is a complex process governed by a variety of mechanisms covering a wide range of cytokines, molecules and immune cells and is triggered by a range of entities such as microbes, exogenous particles and even some endogenous proteins and fatty acids. The non-microbial inflammation is one of the major mechanisms induced in obesity and diabetes mellitus. It has been noted that the expression of a few inflammatory markers gets elevated in metabolic pathological conditions. Some of the most potent inflammatory proteins such as TNF-α, IL-6, IL-1β, IL-8, CRP and receptors such as TLR-2 and TLR-4 have accelerated expression in hyperglycaemia. Apart from the release of these cytokines, the most important cell mediated inflammatory reaction associated with diabetes and obesity is the classical activation of macrophages by saturated free fatty acids. These activated macrophages are more prone to attaching onto endothelial cells, engulfing circulating lipids to become foam cells and initiating the concerned inflammatory reactions. As it is said that nature has everything to sustain life on this planet, every deleterious effect would definitely be countered by its antagonistic beneficial phenomenon. A few studies on anti-inflammatory cytokines such as IL-10 and IL-13 have shown that administration of IL-13 can attenuate the diabetic inflammatory reactions and can bring back the normoglycaemic state. Anti-TNF-α antibodies have been shown to have great anti-hyperglycaemic activity in animal models as well as human subjects. A large systematic meta-analysis (19,709 participants for IL-6 and 40,735 participants for CRP) of the relation between T2DM and the two inflammatory markers IL-6 and CRP revealed that there is a direct positive correlation between the two markers and incidence of T2DM. This large meta-analysis also proposed, as with previous studies, that chronic inflammation could be a valuable predictor of T2DM development risk. IL-6 may interact and hamper the insulin signalling pathway in β-cells. By helping in the production of CRP, this study postulates that IL-6, as compared to CRP, is a stronger predictor of T2DM, and CRP is more of a downstream protein of T2DM than a causal factor [25]. Donath et al. reviewed the relation between inflammation and diabetes and reported that certain major factors responsible for the occurrence of diabetes are glucotoxicity (high blood sugar hampers β-cell and may lead to their death), lipotoxicity (long chain fatty acids in plasma in obese individuals also results in β-cell damage and death), oxidative stress (high blood glucose results in oxidative stress that is particularly detrimental to β-cells since they scarcely have protective antioxidants), endoplasmic reticulum stress (results from insulin resistant state) and possibly islet amyloid deposition in the β-cells. Hypoxia has readily been observed in pathologically rapidly growing cells such as adipocytes in obese condition. The hypoxic condition results in the recruitment of large amounts of macrophages around the cells and initiates the inflammatory response in obese condition. Macrophages also surround the cells that have died due to increased hypoxia, further leading to the release of pro-inflammatory mediators [26]. Thus, these pro-inflammatory cytokine inhibition and anti-inflammatory cytokine elevation or administration could serve as promising projected therapeutic approaches against diabetes and associated inflammation-induced deleterious effects.

REFERENCES

1. Shoelson SE, Lee J, Goldfine AB. Inflammation and insulin resistance. *J Clin Invest* 2006;116(7):1793–1801.
2. Badawi A, Klip A, Haddad P, Cole DEC, Bailo BG. Type 2 diabetes mellitus and inflammation: Prospects for biomarkers of risk and nutritional intervention. *Diab Metab Syn Obes Target Ther* 2010;3:173–186.
3. Hotamisligil GS, Shargill NS, Spiegelman BM. Adipose expression of tumor necrosis factor-α: Direct role in obesity-linked insulin resistance. *Science* 1993;259(5091):87–91.
4. Chawla A, Nguyen KD, Goh YPS. Macrophage-mediated inflammation in metabolic disease. *Nat Rev Immunol* 2012;11(11):738–749.
5. Odegaard JI, Chawla A. Alternative macrophage activation and metabolism. *Annu Rev Pathol* 2012;6:275–297.
6. Dasu MR, Devaraj S, Zhao L, Hwang DH, Jialal I. High glucose induces toll-like receptor expression in human monocytes mechanism of activation. *Diabetes* 2008;57(11):3090–3098.
7. Gacka M, Dobosz T, Szymaniec S, Chabowska DB, Adamiec R, Sadakierska-Chudy A. Proinflammatory and atherogenic activity of monocytes in Type 2 diabetes. *J Diabetes Complications* 2010;24(1):1–8.
8. Hotamisligil GS, Murray DL, Choy LN, Spiegelman BM. Tumor necrosis factor a inhibits signaling from the insulin receptor. *Proc Natl Acad Sci USA* 1994;91(11):4854–4858.
9. Hotamisligil GS, Spiegelman BM. Tumor necrosis factor a: A key component of the obesity-diabetes link. *Diabetes* 1994;43(11):1271–1278.
10. Plomgaard P, Neilsen AR, Fischer CP, Mortensen OH, Broholm C. Associations between insulin resistance and TNF-α in plasma, skeletal muscle and adipose tissue in humans with and without type 2 diabetes. *Diabetologia* 2007;50(12):2562–2571.
11. Moller DE. Potential role of TNF-a in the pathogenesis of insulin resistance and Type 2 diabetes. *Trends Endocrinol Metab* 2000;11(6):212–217.
12. Duncan BB, Schmidt MI, Pankow JS, Ballantyne CM, Couper D, Vigo A et al. Low-grade systemic inflammation and the development of type 2 diabetes: The atherosclerosis risk in communities study. *Diabetes* 2003;52(7):1799–1805.
13. Spranger J, Kroke A, Mohlig M, Hoffmann K, Bergmann MM, Ristow M, et al. Inflammatory cytokines and the risk to develop Type 2 diabetes results of the prospective population-based European prospective investigation into cancer and nutrition (EPIC)-Potsdam study. *Diabetes* 2003;52(3):812–817.
14. Banerjee M, Saxena M. Interleukin-1 (IL-1) family of cytokines: Role in type 2 diabetes. *Clin Chim Acta* 2012;413(15–16):1163–1170.
15. Ehses JA, Lacraz G, Giroix MH, Schmidlin F, Coulaud J, Kassis JC et al. IL-1 antagonism reduces hyperglycemia and tissue inflammation in the type 2 diabetic GK rat. *Proc Natl Acad Sci USA* 2009;106(33):13998–14003.
16. Mirza S, Hossain M, Mathews C, Martinez P, Pino P, Gay JL et al. Type 2-diabetes is associated with elevated levels of TNF-alpha, IL-6 and adiponectin and low levels of leptin in a population of Mexican Americans: A cross-sectional study. *Cytokine* 2012;57(1):136–142.
17. Honkanen J, Nieminen JK, Gao R, Luopajarvi K, Salo H, Ilonen J et al. IL-17 immunity in human Type 1 diabetes. *J Immunol* 2010;185(3):1959–1967.
18. Li S, Joseph C, Becourt C, Klibi J, Luce S, Dubois-Laforgue D et al. Potential role of IL-17-producing iNKT cells in type 1 diabetes. *PLoS One* 2014;9(4):e96151.

19. Pradhan AD, Manson JE, Rifai N, Buring JE, Ridker PM. C-reactive protein, interleukin-6, and risk of developing type 2 diabetes mellitus. *JAMA* 2001;286(3):327–334.
20. Bastard JP, Maachi M, Lagathu C, Kim MJ, Caron M, Vidal H et al. Recent advances in the relationship between obesity inflammation, and insulin resistance. *Eur Cytokine Netw* 2006;17(1):4–12.
21. Badawi A, Klip A, Haddad P, Cole DE, Bailo B, El-Sohemy A et al. Type 2 diabetes mellitus and inflammation: Prospects for biomarkers of risk and nutritional intervention. *Diab Metab Synd Obes Target Ther* 2010;3:173–186.
22. Pickup JC. Inflammation and activated innate immunity in the pathogenesis of Type 2 diabetes. *Diabetes Care* 2004;27(3):813–823.
23. Devaraj S, Glaser N, Griffen S, Wang-Polagruto J, Miguelino E, Jialal I. Increased monocytic activity and biomarkers of inflammation in patients with type 1 diabetes. *Diabetes* 2006;55(3):774–779.
24. Dasu MR, Park S, Devaraj S, Jialal I. Increased toll-like receptor (TLR) activation and TLR ligands in recently diagnosed type 2 diabetic subjects. *Diabetes Care* 2010;33(4):861–868.
25. Wang X, Bao W, Liu J, Ouyang YY, Wang D, Rong S et al. Inflammatory markers and risk of type 2 diabetes: A systematic review and meta-analysis. *Diabetes Care* 2013;36(1):166–175.
26. Donath MY, Shoelson SE. Type 2 diabetes as an inflammatory disease. *Nat Rev Immunol* 2011;11(2):98–10.

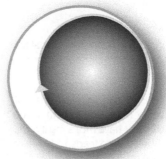

3 Insulin Resistance and Glucose Regulation

INTRODUCTION TO INSULIN RESISTANCE

Diabetes mellitus is a collective term used for a plethora of diseases characterised primarily by hyperglycaemia. Uncontrolled hyperglycaemia, and thus diabetes, leads to a wide array of metabolic pathological conditions such as cardiovascular disorders (CVD), retinopathy, nephropathy, hepatic dysfunction and many more. The World Health Organization (WHO) and Centres for Disease Control and Prevention (CDC) state that among all the forms of diabetes, type 2 diabetes or non-insulin dependent diabetes mellitus (T2DM) is the most common and the risk of death due to CVD and stroke is two to four times greater in diabetic individuals with uncontrolled hyperglycaemia as compared to non-diabetic individuals [1]. Insulin resistance (IRes) is a pathological condition where the target tissue become unresponsiveness to the exposed amount of insulin and thus cannot store and utilise the glucose effectively. The physiological role of insulin is to store glucose in the form of triglycerides in adipocytes and glycogen in the liver and skeletal muscles. The body thus encounters hyperinsulinaemia (around a two-fold increase in basal insulin level) and hyperglycaemia too. Continuous insulin exposure also leads to a reduction in the number of insulin receptors (IR) on the target cells by enhancing receptor internalisation and degradation [2]. Insulin resistance and resultant compensatory hyperinsulinaemia may not cause sudden hyperglycaemia but greatly increase the risk of hypertriglyceridaemia, low high-density lipoprotein (HDL) and essential hypertension (HTN). These conditions may significantly increase the risk of CVD if not controlled [3]. Obesity is one of the major culprits for type 2 diabetes where insulin resistance is the primary link. Obese people were shown to have decreased insulin responsive glucose transporter GLUT-4 on adipocytes and even their skeletal muscle cells were devoid of proper insulin signalling. Hypertrophied adipocytes tend to release more fatty acids in circulation (free fatty acids or FFA) and this excess FFA has been shown to be a major factor in diminished insulin signalling [4]. It has been reported that a high-fat diet (HFD) in mice resulted in attenuation of glucose stimulated insulin secretion (GSIS) from pancreatic β-cells by reducing the expression of GLUT-2 receptor on β-cells which in turn reduces the uptake of glucose from blood. HFD also resulted in glucose intolerance, insulin resistance, hepatic steatosis and body weight gain. In muscle cells, the insulin resistance results in decreased glucose uptake while hepatic insulin resistance results in suppression of gluconeogenesis but retains the insulin-stimulated lipogenesis [5, 6].

It was reported in 1997 that free fatty acids (FFA) or non-esterified fatty acids (NEFA) are one of the strongest links between obesity and insulin resistance, eventually leading to type 2 diabetes. Plasma FFA has been shown to be elevated in most obese individuals. This elevated plasma FFA hinders the insulin facilitated glucose transport in the target cells

[7, 8]. Apart from plasma FFA, another factor of obesity responsible for insulin resistance is body mass index (BMI). It has been observed that people with more central or abdominal obesity have more insulin resistance as compared to those with more peripheral fat. Obesity also leads to β-cell dysfunction and thus hampered insulin secretion [9]. One of the important aspects of insulin resistance is its effect on and through the liver. Insulin normally suppresses hepatic glucose production but this effect is reduced in the case of hepatic insulin resistance. This results in excessive hepatic glucose production and eventual hyperglycaemia. In a high-fat diet fed state, hepatic insulin resistance is the first to occur, and then resistance in other insulin responsive tissue occurs. Hyperglycaemia and hyperinsulinaemia finally lead to parenchymal lipid deposition in the liver, resulting in hepatic steatosis [10].

Another important feature of adipocytes involved in insulin sensitivity and insulin resistance is the special biological protein/peptide messengers secreted from them known as 'adipocytokines' or more accurately 'adipokines'. The molecules are basically regulatory and inflammatory. They play an important part in energy and vascular homeostasis. The major studied adipokines are namely leptin, adiponectin, resistin, visfatin, TNF-α and others. Adiponectin has been shown to increase insulin sensitivity; even the anti-diabetic medicines of the thiazolidinedione (TZD) class increase insulin sensitivity and also increase the expression of adiponectin. Resistin, on the other hand, has been one of the most controversial molecules in view of its action-enhancing insulin resistance (it has been named for the word *resistance*). Few reports also suggest that resistin is not involved in insulin resistance in humans [11]. Ceramide or the precursor of sphingolipid theory is another important aspect which is incremental in insulin resistance. Ceramides require saturated fatty acids for their formation and thus they represent a good candidate relating to insulin resistance since saturated fats accumulate more easily than their unsaturated

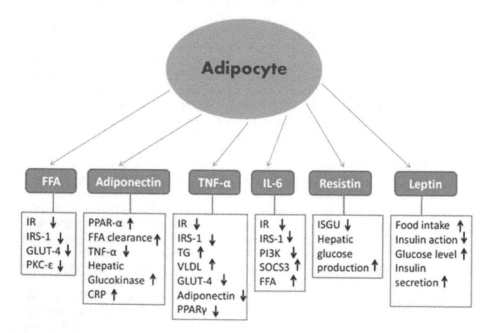

Figure 3.1 Adipokines in insulin resistance.

counterparts and tend to deposit more, causing insulin resistance. Ceramides are also imbibed in blood through the dietary sphingolipids which get degraded to generate the former. It has also been reported that ceramides inhibit the insulin-stimulated glucose uptake, GLUT-4 translocation on the cell surface, and glycogen synthesis in the insulin-responsive muscle cells. It was also seen that ceramide-induced insulin resistance is more pronounced in skeletal muscle cells [12]. The following sections describe in detail the various factors and related mechanisms involved in one of the major causes of metabolic worry throughout the globe, i.e. insulin resistance (Figure 3.1).

OBESITY AS A CAUSE OF INSULIN RESISTANCE

Obesity is well-known factor which results in the development of a serious pathologic outcome known as insulin resistance (IRes). Insulin resistance, in the long run, has been shown to increase the risk of development of T2DM, which itself is the disease known for its ability to eventually destroy many organs if not controlled properly. Obesity is the condition of hypertrophy of adipocytes which is the increase in the size of these fat cells due to the increment in the amount of stored triglyceride (TG). The hypertrophied adipocytes play a central role in many pathological conditions, one major one being insulin resistance, where many molecular messengers act as mediators such as FFA, adiponectin, TNF-α, interleukin-6, resistin and others [4, 7]. The WHO recommended that metabolic syndrome should be diagnosed with insulin resistance markers along with any two markers among obesity, hypertension, hypertriglyceridaemia, low high-density lipoproteins (HDL) level and hypercholesterolaemia. The National Cholesterol Education Program Adult Treatment Panel III (ATP III) recommended in 2001 that three of the following five factors should be present to show the presence of metabolic syndrome: Abdominal obesity (major factor for IRes), hypertriglyceridaemia, reduced HDL, hypertension and elevated fasting blood glucose. The International Diabetes Federation (IDF), in 2005, said that abdominal obesity, with special emphasis on waist measurement, should be one of the essential requirements for metabolic syndrome. The American Heart Association (AHA) also emphasised that the threshold for waist measurement to give rise to metabolic syndrome in the European population should be $\geq$102 cm (in males) and $\geq$88 cm (in females), which correspond to a body mass index (BMI) of 30 kg/m². BMI is defined as the ratio of body mass (in kg) to the height of person (in m²) and is regarded as one of the major criteria for defining the obese state. But the discrepancy lies in the fact that different ethnic populations have different genetic predispositions towards height and weight and thus an Indian with a certain BMI may be regarded as overweight, while a European with same BMI may not be overweight. Thus waist circumference is generally received better than BMI [13]. We will briefly review some of the major messenger molecules released from hypertrophied adipocytes and related inflammatory cells responsible for insulin resistance.

Free Fatty Acids

Boden (1994) stated that free fatty acids (FFA) or non-esterified fatty acids (NEFA) are one of the biggest culprits for inducing insulin resistance. He showed that FFA level is increased in most of the obese subjects which in turn inhibit the insulin-stimulated peripheral glucose uptake. Apart from inhibition of glucose uptake, he also experimentally proposed that glucose phosphorylation as well as glycogen synthase activity in skeletal muscle cells are also hampered by antagonising the insulin action. He also speculated that elevated FFA results in overstimulation of hepatic glucose production, resulting in continuous elevated plasma glucose [14]. Roden (1996) also elaborated the fact through his experimental observation that elevated plasma FFA causes insulin resistance by inhibition of glucose transport and its further phosphorylation with reduction in the rate of glycogen synthesis in muscles [15]. Insulin resistance has been the major cause of T2DM, other than the genetic predisposition towards it. Obesity has long since been considered as one of the major causes of insulin resistance and it has been observed that weight reduction increases the insulin sensitivity in the target tissues.

Insulin receptor substrate (IRS-1 and IRS-2) proteins are the major proteins directly attached to the IR and convey the signalling cascade further. In a simple explanation of insulin action, insulin binds to the IR present on the cell membrane. The IR gets autophosphorylated at tyrosine residues and further activates IRS-1 and IRS-2. These proteins further activate PI-3 kinase and finally Akt/PKB. Akt finally activates and recruits GLUT-4 (the primary insulin responsive glucose transporter) on the cell membrane so that it can bring the circulating glucose inside the cell. Free fatty acids are seen to become stored in non-adipose cells, leading to increased intramyocellular lipid depots, and leading to insulin resistance. It has also been shown that FFA-induced insulin resistance is related to downregulation of the insulin receptor (IR) gene. FFA also inhibits the activation of PI-3 kinase in the skeletal muscle cells. It has also been found that saturated fats block the insulin activation of Akt/PKB signalling. These FFA inhibitory actions finally result in diminished GLUT-4 translocation to membranes, finally increasing the plasma glucose [16]. FFAs also serve as a great substrate for hepatic TG synthesis and hepatic gluconeogenesis which results in elevated plasma VLDL and hyperglycaemia.

Reduction in IR expression has further been stated in obese mice models with hepatic steatosis. Further, it has been found that saturated fatty acids reduce the mRNA and protein level of IR in cell lines of hepatocyte and skeletal muscle. Some reports also suggest that IR expression is inversely related to protein kinase C (PKCε isoform) in obese animal models. PKCε has been found to impair the HMGA1 which is the major transcription factor of the IR gene. In a breakthrough study, it was reported that lipids phosphorylate PKCε through palmitoylation. Phosphorylated PKCε in turn impairs HMGA1 which finally reduces the IR expression leading to a significant decrease in insulin sensitivity [17].

Adiponectin

Adiponectin is a 30 kDa protein mainly produced from mature adipocytes. It is present in systemic circulation as trimer, hexamer and 12–18mer. The physiological plasma concentration in humans ranges from 5–30 µg/ml. It is probably the only adipokine which is negatively related to obesity, diabetes and related complications. The two major receptors for adiponectin are AdipoR1 and AdipoR2. The former is highly expressed in skeletal muscle cells while the latter is primarily expressed in hepatocytes. Binding of adiponectin to its receptors results in insulin sensitising and 'fat-burning' effects, while also possessing anti-atherogenic, anti-inflammatory and anti-oxidant properties. The insulin-sensitising effect of adiponectin is mediated through a variety of actions such as reduction in hepatic gluconeogenesis, increase in muscle glucose transport, enhancement of fatty acid oxidation in hepatocytes and muscle cells, reduced plasma triglyceride and increased VLDL catabolism. Adiponectin also attenuates TNF-α expression and related inflammatory processes improving overall insulin sensitivity in the target tissues [18].

It was demonstrated in many animal studies that the adiponectin mRNA expression and adiponectin plasma concentration decreased in the animal models of obesity. The level of adiponectin was also found to be decreased in monkeys who were fed with a high-fat diet, leading to insulin resistance and finally T2DM [19]. Maeda et al. found that adiponectin knock-out (KO) mice displayed delayed plasma FFA clearance, low fatty-acid transport protein 1 in skeletal muscle cells, high TNF-α mRNA expression in adipocytes and high plasma concentration of TNF-α. The adiponectin KO mice also displayed severe insulin resistance when fed with a high-fat diet due to decreased IRS-1 mediated PI-3 kinase signalling in muscle cells [20]. Clinically, too, the adiponectin was found to be decreased drastically in obese individuals as compared to the lean subjects, and thus negatively correlated with body mass index (BMI). In another important study, it was found that plasma adiponectin was much less in diabetic subjects as compared to the non-diabetics and even further decreased in patients who had diabetes as well as coronary artery disease. It was also found that adiponectin was inversely correlated to the lipid profile, especially plasma triglyceride [21].

Pharmacologically, too, the activation of peroxisome proliferator activated receptor-γ (PPAR-γ) by the thiazolidinedione (TZDs) class of anti-diabetic results in an increase in the plasma adiponectin level, contributing to the insulin-sensitising effect of TZDs [22]. Mouse models of obesity and insulin resistance also displayed significantly lower expression of AdipoR1 and AdipoR2. Hepatic expression of AdipoR2 in animal models demonstrated increased expression of genes such as glucokinase (involved in hepatic glucose uptake) and PPAR-α. Further activation of AMP activated protein kinase (AMPK) resulted in a reduction in endogenous hepatic glucose production. Expression of both AdipoR1 and AdipoR2 resulted in increased fatty acid oxidation, decreased hepatic TG content and thus improved insulin sensitivity. Conversely, deactivation of both of the receptors resulted in high hepatic and plasma TG and significantly increased insulin resistance [23]. The adiponectin level was found to be decreased by increased plasma TNF-α in obesity. These two molecules, thus, have an inverse correlation. The common inflammatory molecule C-reactive protein (CRP), which is increased in obesity, is also inversely correlated with the level of adiponectin [24].

Adiponectin, on binding to its receptors, initiates a range of signalling cascade mainly activating AMPK, mTOR, NF-κB, STAT3 and JNK. AMPK phosphorylation results in increased glucose uptake by skeletal muscle cells and reduced hepatic gluconeogenesis. The adipokines also enhance nitric oxide (NO) production by activating endothelial nitric oxide synthase (eNOS), showing positive vascular effects [25]. In another major experimental study, it was found that adiponectin and HDL were positively correlated and negatively with insulin resistance. Thus, with an increasing incidence of childhood obesity, it is evident that a continuous decrease in adiponectin may result in insulin resistance and eventually T2DM and atherogenic conditions [26].

TNF-α

In 1993, Hotamisligil et al. demonstrated that TNF-α mRNA expression in mature adipocytes was increased in animal models of obesity and diabetes. The plasma level of TNF-α was also significantly elevated and this level was directly related to the intensity of insulin resistance, while inhibition of the molecule resulted in increased peripheral insulin-stimulated glucose uptake [27]. It was also demonstrated in another important study that TNF-α decreased the insulin-stimulated IR autophosphorylation and the corresponding resulting phosphorylation of IRS-1. The structure–function relationship of the isolated IR from the TNF-α treated cells was also significantly disturbed. These results showed that TNF-α was directly responsible for downregulation of insulin signalling, giving rise to insulin resistance. It was also reported that the tyrosine phosphorylation of IRS-1 is also reduced in adipocytes and skeletal muscle cells due to TNF-α leading to insulin resistant state [28]. *In vivo* TNF-α administration also resulted in elevated plasma TG and VLDL mainly due to increased hepatic lipogenesis. Another major effect of the molecule is the inhibition of GLUT-4 expression in adipocytes and marked decrease in glucose uptake in muscle cells [29].

It was also evident in animal studies that the absence of TNF-α or TNF-α receptors resulted in improved insulin sensitivity in animal models of obesity and diabetes. The cytokine was also shown to increase the adipocytes lipolysis, resulting in elevated plasma FFA; again gaining cycle of FFA-induced insulin resistance. TNF-α was also shown to downregulate the expression of proteins involved in energy and lipid homeostasis such as adiponectin, GLUT-4, IRS-1 and PPARγ in adipocytes. In another important manner, TNF-α activates NF-κB which in turn decreases the expression of PPARγ, resulting in insulin resistance [30]. In another important study in the search for further mechanism for TNF-α mediated insulin resistance, it was found that TNF-α modulates IR signalling through activation of the protein tyrosine phosphatase (PTP) enzyme, which reverses the tyrosine phosphorylation in IR signalling. In the same study, the scientists found that prolonged hyperglycaemia inhibits IR signalling by activating PKC [31].

Resistin and Interleukin-6

Resistin is a 12 kDa adipocyte-derived polypeptide. It is expressed and secreted not only by mature adipocytes but also expressed in macrophages in a much higher amount. It was named due to the fact that it was believed to be linked directly to insulin resistance. Resistin is perhaps the most controversial adipokine since many researchers supported the fact that it induces insulin resistance in animal models of obesity and diabetes but those working with human cells or subjects directly deny the fact. In an early breakthrough study published in 2001, researchers showed, using animal models and mouse adipocytes cell line, that resistin is the link between obesity and diabetes [32]. But, in fact, many human studies failed to link resistin to insulin resistance and it is even said that it is the adipose tissue macrophage rather than the human adipocytes that produce resistin [33].

Mice models with obesity and diabetes induced by a high-fat diet showed elevated serum resistin and reduced insulin sensitivity, while administration of the anti-resistin antibody to the same animal improved the insulin sensitivity. Even the administration of recombinant resistin to normal mice resulted in insulin resistance. Resistin also inhibited the insulin-stimulated glucose uptake (ISGU) in the cultured 3T3-L1 mouse adipocytes, while its infusion in normal rat resulted in increased hepatic insulin resistance and hepatic glucose production. Its production from macrophages was also supported by the fact that its mRNA level was found to be very low in obese mice, but serum concentration was significantly elevated and related to insulin resistance. In contrast to the animal studies, the human studies demonstrate that human adipocytes do not produce resistin; rather, it is the adipose stromal macrophages which produce resistin [33, 34].

Interleukin-6 (IL-6) is a cytokine produced by a variety of cells such as immune cells, endothelial cells and fibroblasts. It is a 22–27 kDa pro-inflammatory protein which binds to its transmembrane receptor gp130. Approximately 30% of IL-6 is secreted by adipocytes; thus, it has been listed as an important adipokine. Like many adipokines, IL-6 level has been positively correlated to insulin resistance and T2DM. It has been seen that weight reduction decreases the IL-6 concentration, thereby improving insulin sensitivity. Among the many mechanisms involved in developing insulin resistance, IL-6 decreases IRS-1 activation, and the PI-3 kinase is decreased while hepatic glycogenesis is also significantly reduced, indicating a hepatic insulin resistance as well. The decrease in IR and IRS-1 phosphorylation is subjected to the fact that IL-6 upregulates SOCS3 expression which in turn displays such actions. Infusion of recombinant IL-6 in animal models also resulted in elevated hepatic glucose production. It also has a marked action of increasing FFA which also augments the insulin resistance. It also partly downregulates the expression of adiponectin. TNF-α is also said to induce the expression of IL-6. An important controversy lies in the fact that IL-6 promotes FFA oxidation and promotes uptake of glucose in skeletal muscle cells [34–36], while reducing the hepatic glycogenesis and glucose uptake in adipocytes, with the mechanisms remaining unclear.

Leptin

The leptin gene (*ob*) was discovered in 1994 by Friedman et al. and it was found that a mutation in this gene leads to obesity [37]. Leptin, a 16 kDa protein hormone, was one of the earliest adipokines discovered that is involved in regulating the food intake and thus the satiety signal. Binding of leptin to neuronal leptin receptors leads to lowering of food intake. Besides this, it is also involved in energy expenditure, body weight regulation and neuro-endocrine activities. In contrast to the above statement, obese human models have been found to have hyperleptinaemia which is a result of leptin resistance. Leptin also has a strong peripheral action, especially on skeletal muscle cells, and is also involved in insulin secretion. Elevated glucose and insulin increases the leptin concentration. This, in turn, is involved in increasing peripheral insulin sensitivity and decreases insulin secretion from pancreatic β-cells. Leptin increases glucose uptake and oxidation in skeletal muscle cells. Leptin also suppresses hepatic output, thus inhibiting an unnecessary rise in glucose level [38]. The research says that insulin and leptin levels have a strong positive correlation, i.e. insulin-sensitive people have lower circulating leptin, while those with insulin resistance (high fasting plasma insulin) have higher leptin concentration, and this relation is independent of body fat mass. This fact is also supported by the fact that obese people have higher leptin levels (leptin resistance) and frequently low insulin resistance. Zimmet et al. found that insulin resistance (higher plasma fasting insulin) is associated with elevated leptin concentration which is independent of body mass distribution, adiposity and gender. It was also reported that leptin level, corresponding to that found in obesity when administered, antagonised insulin signalling. This might lead to the fact that increased leptin secretion with increased adiposity (obesity) may be one of the factors behind insulin resistance [39]. Leptin knock-out mice were shown to develop hyperglycaemia, hyperinsulinaemia and insulin resistance, while leptin treatment reversed these metabolic symptoms. Leptin administration in normally fed mice resulted in decreased plasma insulin and associated glucose elevation. Leptin, thus, reduces insulin secretion. This reduction in insulin secretion is also supposed to be mediated by the action of leptin on specific leptin receptors present on the insulin-producing beta-cells of pancreas affecting the PLC/PKC mediated insulin releasing pathway. Another probable mechanism proposed is the activation of the phosphodiesterase 3B enzyme leading to suppression of GLP-1 mediated insulin release. Apart from the effect on insulin secretion, leptin also modifies the insulin action. Leptin infusion in rats resulted in increased hepatic and peripheral insulin sensitivity. The effect was more profound in peripheral sensitivity [40].

Leptin deficiency by birth (congenital) has been associated with hyperphagia, insulin resistance, hyperlipidaemia and impaired thermogenesis. Leptin directly suppresses appetite by inhibiting the orexigenic peptides neuropeptide Y (NPY) and agouti-related peptide (AgRP). Leptin also activates PI3K which is an important mechanism regulating glucose uptake by insulin signalling. Leptin has also been shown to activate AMPK, thus limiting the accumulation of triglycerides in hepatocytes and skeletal muscle cells, resulting in improved insulin signalling. Attenuation of leptin signalling at neuronal leptin receptors leads to increased accumulation of triglyceride in adipocytes, hepatocytes and skeletal muscle cells, resulting in insulin resistance at these major sites [41]. Leptin, in physiological amount, protects the peripheral skeletal muscle cells from lipotoxicity, but hyperleptinaemia leads to leptin resistance. Thus, a high leptin level or leptin resistance would not show its protective effects of a decreasing cellular lipid store and increasing insulin sensitivity, but rather would increase insulin resistance.

FIBROBLAST GROWTH FACTOR 21

Another important recent marker proposed that has shown considerable association with insulin resistance and diabetes is a new member of the fibroblast growth factor family – FGF21. Fibroblast growth factors (FGFs) are a class of glycoproteins responsible mainly for growth and metabolism. FGFs are autocrine, paracrine or endocrine in their action. Endocrine FGFs mainly work like hormone and affect metabolism. The human FGF family consists of 22 members with the majority functioning in growth, development and cellular differentiation, but the FGF19 subfamily members, comprising FGF15/19, FGF21 and FGF23, exert metabolic effect by endocrine action. While most other FGFs show their FGF receptor (FGFR) binding through binding to heparin sulphate of extracellular matrix (ECM), FGF21 binds to heparin sulphate very weakly and thus works in an endocrine manner. Another important feature of FGF21 activity is that the FGFRs that it binds to are combined to another transmembrane protein β-klotho which is primarily expressed in adipocytes, hepatocytes and the pancreas. Thus these organs are the major sites of action of FGF21. Thus, from the sites of action, it becomes apparent that FGF21 is involved in lipid, glucose and bile acid metabolism [42].

In initial experiments with cultured mouse and human adipocytes, it was found that FGF21 facilitated glucose uptake in these cells independent of insulin through expression of GLUT-1 receptors. Administration of recombinant FGF21 to diabetic and obese animal models resulted in lowering of plasma glucose, improved insulin sensitivity and decreased lipid parameters gained due to the highly fed diet [43]. While physiological levels of FGF21 show a positive metabolic effect on carbohydrate and lipid metabolism, it has been shown that FGF21 level is increased significantly in the case of obesity (increased adiposity) and is positively correlated with insulin resistance. This implies that a high FGF21 in obesity leads to a FGF21-resistant state where it cannot perform its physiological activity. It was also found that subjects with MS had a significantly higher level of FGF21 as compared to those who did not show MS. Moreover, the protein was independently associated with the MS and thus could be used as a potential biomarker for it [44].

There is evidence that administration of FGF21 attenuates several obesity-induced metabolic parameters such as high plasma glucose and plasma FFA, but it is also a contradictory fact that obese people have high circulating FGF21 which clearly states that it has a tendency similar to hyperinsulinaemia and hyperleptinaemia in obese subjects. Contradictory to this, data from an experimental study shows that FGF21 administration in obese mice was not as effective in reducing glucose as compared to the effect in lean mice. This was due to impaired induction of GLUT-1 in response to FGF21 in obese mice. Expression of FGF receptors was also shown to be reduced in the liver in obesity, which is quite similar to the downregulation of insulin receptors in obese models [45]. Human studies in a clinical follow-up by the Baltimore Longitudinal Study of Aging (BLSA) also indicate that higher FGF21 was associated with obesity and dyslipidaemia and is an independent risk factor of type 2 diabetes or T2DM. Elevated FGF21 was also associated independently with insulin resistance, showing a positive correlation with insulin resistance [46]. These and several other studies indicate that obesity certainly exhibits a FGF21-resistant state where the circulating FGF21 is very high but cannot show its beneficial action [47]. Another early study related to this novel hormone demonstrates that FGF21 is positively correlated with an insulin-resistant state and thus it is inversely correlated to both the hepatic and the peripheral insulin sensitivity. But it is still not very apparent that this elevated FGF21 is compensating the insulin-resistant state or is a reason behind the insulin resistance [48].

DIETARY EFFECT ON INSULIN RESISTANCE

Fatty Acid Mediated Insulin Resistance

A common perception and fact is that the regular consumption of a high-fat diet results in diet-induced obesity. High fat intake is also said to be a cause of T2DM, independent of obesity. This risk is subjected to the type of fatty acids consumed in the diet. The fatty acid composition of skeletal muscle cells varies with the change in dietary fatty acids. It was shown long ago that T2DM patients had a greater amount of saturated fatty acids in their plasma as compared to non-diabetic subjects, who had more linoleic acid. The insulin sensitivity of skeletal muscle cells was directly proportional to the amount of long-chain polyunsaturated fatty acids in the cell membrane [36]. The replacement of safflower oil with fish oil (rich in omega-3 fatty acids) in a rat diet prevented the development of insulin resistance in hepatocytes and skeletal muscle cells. Diets rich in saturated fats result in elevated TG in hepatocytes. In a breakthrough study, it was found that skeletal muscle insulin resistance was directly related to the amount of triglyceride accumulation in those cells, while the percentage of long chain omega-3 fatty acids was directly related to the insulin stimulated glucose uptake; omega-6 fatty acid rich diets were also involved in stimulating insulin resistance [49].

It was seen that high-fat diets in rats and mice resulted in the accumulation of TG and ceramide in muscles, leading to the activation of NF-κB, which resulted in diminished insulin action. Saturated fatty acids, in particular, have been shown to initiate TLR-2 and TLR-4 (toll-like receptor) mediated inflammatory reactions, leading to poor insulin sensitivity. A high-carbohydrate diet was shown to increase the expression and release of inflammatory IL-6 and expression of TLR-2 and TLR-4 [50]. Among different edible categories, foods with a high glycaemic index rating were associated with declining insulin sensitivity. Fructose intake was well-associated with hepatic insulin resistance, but not peripheral insulin resistance. A saturated fatty acid rich diet was associated with significant decrease in insulin sensitivity as compared to an unsaturated fatty acid diet, as found in a large human study [50]. Storlein et al. have shown that the replacement of omega-6 fatty acids with omega-3 fatty acids in the diet is capable of attenuating the insulin resistance developed from the high-fructose diet in the rat model. The same strategy was applicable and useful in humans too [51]. Interestingly, it was shown that high saturated fat diet resulted in a defect in GLUT-4 membrane translocation and thus resulted in insulin resistance even when GLUT-4 is expressed normally. In another important study by Shullman et al., it was shown that fatty acid activates protein kinase C (PKC). PKC activation resulted in serine/threonine phosphorylation of IRS, inhibiting the physiological tyrosine phosphorylation and thus damaging the insulin signalling pathway and promoting insulin resistance [52, 53].

Fatty acid type and composition plays a significant role in metabolic diseases, especially diabetes and obesity. Though still a matter of debate and research, but it is evident through various reliable scientific articles that increase omega-6 fatty acids and saturated fatty acids can be pro-inflammatory in nature while omega-3 fatty acids (primarily eicosapentaenoic acid or EPA and docosahexaenoic acid or DHA) have beneficial effects over inflammatory conditions [54]. There have been lots of research on the metabolic effects of these fatty acids. In a recent meta-analysis by de Souza et al. [55], it was pointed out that intake of saturated fat was not related to all cause mortality, cardiovascular diseases, coronary heart disease, and type 2 diabetes. It was the trans-fat that has harmful effects on human system. Though, large consumption of saturated fats could impair insulin sensitivity. In another meta-analysis by Aune et al., [56] an inverse relationship was observed between dairy product intake and type 2 diabetes. The analysis included effects of milk, yogurt, cheese, and cottage cheese as major dairy food sources. As mentioned above, omega-6 polyunsaturated fatty acids (PUFA) have been considered to be pro-inflammatory, the ratio of omega-6 and omega-3 is considered an essential factor in dietary fat consumption. In a recent well-reviewed article, it has been mentioned that consumption of linoleic acid (LA; omega-6 PUFA) containing seed oils contributes to low-grade inflammation, oxidative stress, and endothelial dysfunction that are strong causative factors for atherosclerosis. Another major fact mentioned was that consumption of LA results in elevated expression of cyclooxygenase-2 in aorta that results in increased breakdown of arachidonic acid into pro-inflammatory eicosanoids. LA also increases the pro-inflammatory conditions in endothelial cells that could contribute to coronary heart disease. On the other hand, edible fats rich in omega-3 fatty acids are shown to reduce inflammation by reducing the levels of inflammatory cytokines. The anti-inflammatory action of omega-3 fatty acids have been well documented in a recent REDUCE-IT trial [57].

The metabolic effects of dietary fatty acids are highly regulated by their physical state too, most importantly whether they are oxidized or not. This oxidation (or hydrolysis) is known as rancidification. As a basic chemistry, saturated fats are very less prone to oxidation compared to the unsaturated fats. Oxidation of edible oils can generate toxic compounds and oxidized polymers [58]. Though omega-3 PUFA is considered to have anti-inflammatory response, it exerts the action in its normal state. Omega-3 PUFA are highly prone to peroxidation that results in cytotoxic compounds where 4-hydroxy-2-alkenals are the primary compounds. These compounds have also been reported to have genotoxicity [59]. The harmful products generated after edible oil rancidification are considered pro-inflammatory and can lead to metabolic diseases and cancer.

Fructose-Induced Insulin Resistance

In a groundbreaking study back in 1987 by Hwang et al., it was shown that rats fed with a fructose-rich diet developed significant hypertension along with hyperinsulinaemia and hypertriglyceridaemia, leading to significant insulin resistance [60]. Thorburn et al. demonstrated the findings on the rat model that a fructose-fed diet was directly responsible for significant insulin resistance and an elevation in plasma triglyceride compared to feeding on glucose or starch [61]. A major study involving nutrient consumption in the United States between 1909 and 1997 found that there was a significant correlation between diabetes and dietary intake of fats, carbohydrates and corn syrup. The use of artificial sweeteners, especially high-fructose corn syrup (HFCS), increased by 86%. Fructose consumption has increased to 85–100 grams per day due to the popular and increased use of HFCS. This high level leads to a marked increase in hepatic lipogenesis and TG accumulation, resulting in reduced insulin sensitivity. Due to the fact that β-cells release insulin only in response to glucose uptake, regular fructose consumption would lead to much less insulin release. Insulin-dependent leptin would then be produced in a lesser amount, decreasing the appetite suppression effect and leading to more eating; in turn, high fructose would enable the liver to form more triglyceride and lipids, leading to increased weight gain and resulting in insulin resistance. A two-week fructose-rich diet in rats demonstrated a decrease in mRNA expression of IR and thus low IR on membranes along with decreased IRS-1 phosphorylation. Fructose has also been said to increase the concentration of advanced glycation end-products (AGEs) and FFA. In the report, fructose was also found to be preferable over other carbohydrates for hepatic and peripheral lipogenesis [61].

Fructose is widely found in fruits and is thus known as fruit sugar. Fructose intake from fruits largely reaches about 15–20 grams per day. This level of fructose is not deleterious for the human system but an increased consumption of HFCS and artificial fructose diets have led to an increase in metabolic syndrome giving rise to 'diabesity'. Even turning down excess fat consumption could not prevent the increase in metabolic syndrome and thus, researchers around the globe found and proposed that marked increase in consumption of HFCS is the leading cause of the syndrome [62].

CONCLUSIONS

Insulin resistance has been found to be the key factor for an overall rise in the incidence of metabolic syndrome. Metabolic syndrome, in large, is characterised by obesity, hyperglycaemia, hyperinsulinaemia, hypertriglyceridaemia and hypertension. Obesity has been discussed to be one of the major causes of insulin resistance globally, as its incidence is at an all-time high. Obesity is the result of excess hypertrophied adipocytes. These adipocytes are the greatest source of adipokines, some of which are related positively, while a few others are related negatively to insulin resistance., For example, adiponectin enhances insulin sensitivity while TNF-α and IL-6 are related to increased insulin resistance. Fatty acid composition of high-fat diets has been a great area of query and research. Saturated fats were found to be bad in the context of insulin resistance, while diets rich in omega-3 FA were found to increase insulin sensitivity. And apart from genetic predisposition to obesity, the increase in the consumption of fructose has been the major reason behind obesity and resultant insulin resistance. It would not be extraneous to say that Buddha emphasised the 'middle path' theory and following that, it is always advisable to continue with a balanced diet.

REFERENCES

1. Kumar A, Bharti SK, Kumar A. Type 2 diabetes mellitus: The concerned complications and target organs. *Apollo Med* 2014;11(3):161–166.
2. Shanik MH, Dankner R, Xu Y, Zick Y, Skrha J, Roth J. Insulin resistance and hyperinsulinemia. Is hyperinsulinemia the cart or the horse? *Diabetes Care* 2008;31(Suppl 2):S262–S268.
3. Reaven GM. The insulin resistance syndrome: Definition and dietary approaches to treatment. *Annu Rev Nutr* 2005;25:391–406.
4. Kahn BB, Flier JS. Obesity and insulin resistance. *J Clin Invest* 2000;106(4):473–481.
5. Thorens B. Of fat, β cells, and diabetes. *Cell Metab* 2011;14(4):439–440.
6. Ohtsubo K, Chen MZ, Olefsky JM, Marth JD. Pathway to diabetes through attenuation of pancreatic beta cell glycosylation and glucose transport. *Nat Med* 2011;17(9):1067–1075.
7. Boden G. Role of fatty acids in the pathogenesis of insulin resistance and T2DM. *Diabetes* 1997;46(1):3–10.
8. Boden G. Free fatty acids, insulin resistance, and type 2 diabetes mellitus. *Proc Assoc Am Physicians* 1999;111(3):241–248.
9. Al-Goblan AS, Al-Alfi MA, Khan MZ. Mechanism linking diabetes mellitus and obesity. *Diabetes Metab Synd Obes Target Ther* 2014;7:587–591.
10. Bazotte RB, Silva LG, Schiavon FPM. Insulin resistance in the liver: Deficiency or excess of insulin? *Cell Cycle* 2014;13(16):2494–2500.
11. Zou C, Shao J. Role of adipocytokines in obesity-associated insulin resistance. *J Nutr Biochem* 2008;19(5):277–286.
12. Summers SA. Ceramides in insulin resistance and lipotoxicity. *Prog Lipid Res* 2006;45(1):42–72.
13. Alberti KG, Eckel RH, Grundy SM, Zimmet PZ, Cleeman JI, Karen A et al. Harmonizing the metabolic syndrome: A joint interim statement of the International Diabetes Federation Task Force on Epidemiology and Prevention; National Heart,

Lung, and Blood Institute; American Heart Association; World Heart Federation; International Atherosclerosis Society; and International Association for the Study of Obesity. *Circulation* 2009;120(16):1640–1645.

14. Boden G, Chen X, Ruiz J, White JV, Rossetti L. Mechanisms of fatty acid-induced inhibition of glucose uptake. *J Clin Invest* 1994;93(6):2438–2446.

15. Roden M, Price TB, Perseghin G, Petersen KF, Rothman DL, Gary W et al. Mechanism of free fatty acid–induced insulin resistance in humans. *J Clin Invest* 1996;97(12):2859–2865.

16. Bhattacharya S, Dey D, Roy SS. Molecular mechanism of insulin resistance. *J Bio Sci* 2007;32(2):405–413.

17. Dasgupta S, Bhattacharya S, Maitra S, Pal D, Majumdar S, Datta A et al. Mechanism of lipid induced insulin resistance: Activated PKC ε is a key regulator. *Biochim Biophys Acta* 2011;1812(4):495–506.

18. Maury E, Brichard SM. Adipokine dysregulation, adipose tissue inflammation and metabolic syndrome. *Mol Cell Endocrinol* 2010;314(1):1–16.

19. Hotta K, Funahashi T, Bodkin NL, Ortmeyer HK, Arita Y, Hansen BC et al. Circulating concentrations of the adipocyte protein adiponectin are decreased in parallel with reduced insulin sensitivity during the progression to type 2 diabetes in rhesus monkeys. *Diabetes* 2001;50(5):1126–1133.

20. Maeda N, Shimomura I, Kishida K, Nishizawa H, Matsuda M, Nagaretani H et al. Diet-induced insulin resistance in mice lacking adiponectin/ACRP30. *Nat Med* 2002;8(7):731–737.

21. Hotta K, Funahashi T, Arita Y, Takahashi M, Matsuda M, Okamoto Y et al. Plasma concentrations of a novel, adipose-specific protein, adiponectin, in type 2 diabetic patients. *Arterioscler Thromb Vasc Biol* 2000;20(6):1595–1599.

22. Haluzik M, Parizkova J, Haluzik MM. Adiponectin and its role in the obesity-induced insulin resistance and related complications. *Physiol Res* 2004;53(2):123–129.

23. Rabe K, Lehrke M, Parhofer KG, Broedl UC. Adipokines and insulin resistance. *Mol Med* 2008;14(11–12):741–751.

24. Whitehead JP, Richards AA, Hickman IJ, Macdonald GA, Prins JB. Adiponectin–a key adipokine in the metabolic syndrome. *Diab Obes Metab* 2006;8(3):264–280.

25. Ziemke F, Mantzoros CS. Adiponectin in insulin resistance: Lessons from translational research. *Am J Clin Nutr* 2010;91(1)(Suppl):258S–61S.

26. Singhal A, Jamieson N, Fewtrell M, Deanfield J, Lucas A, Sattar N. Adiponectin predicts insulin resistance but not endothelial function in young, healthy adolescents. *J Clin Endocrinol Metab* 2005;90(8):4615–4621.

27. Hotamisligil GS, Shargill NS, Spiegelman BM. Adipose expression of tumor necrosis factor alpha: Direct role in obesity linked insulin resistance. *Science* 1993;259(5091):8791.

28. Hotamisligil GS, Murray DL, Choy LN, Spiegelman BM. Tumor necrosis factor a inhibits signaling from the insulin receptor. *Proc Natl Acad Sci USA* 1994;91(11):4854–4858.

29. Hotamisligil GS, Spiegelman BM. Tumor necrosis factor a: A key component of the obesity-diabetes link. *Diabetes* 1994;43(11):1271–1278.

30. Ruan H, Lodish HF. Insulin resistance in adipose tissue: Direct and indirect effects of tumor necrosis factor-α. *Cytokine Growth Factor Rev* 2003;14(5):447–455.

31. Kroder G, Bossenmaier B, Kellerer M, Capp E, Stoyanov B, Mühlhöfer A et al. Tumor necrosis factor-α and hyperglycemia-induced insulin resistance. *J Clin Invest* 1996;97(6):1471–1477.

32. Steppan CM, Bailey ST, Bhat S, Brown EJ, Banerjee RR The hormone resistin links obesity to diabetes. *Nature* 2001;409(6818):307–312.

33. Zou C, Shao J. Role of adipocytokines in obesity-associated insulin resistance. *J Nutr Biochem* 2008;19(5):277–286.
34. Steppan CM, Lazar MA. Resistin and obesity-associated insulin resistance. *Trends Endocrinol Metab* 2002;13(1):18–23.
35. Galic S, Oakhill JS, Steinberg GR. Adipose tissue as an endocrine organ. *Mol Cell Endocrinol* 2010;316(2):129–139.
36. Maury E, Brichard SM. Adipokine dysregulation, adipose tissue inflammation and metabolic syndrome. *Mol Cell Endocrinol* 2010;314(1):1–16.
37. Zhang Y, Proenca R, Maffei M, Barone M, Leopold L, Friedman JM. Positional cloning of the mouse obese gene and its human homologue. *Nature* 1994;372(6505):425–432.
38. Yildiz BO, Haznedaroglu IC. Rethinking leptin and insulin action: Therapeutic opportunities diabetes. *Int J Biochem Cell Biol* 2006;38(5-6):820–830.
39. Zimmet PZ, Collins VR, de Courten MP, Hodge AM, Collier GR, Dowse GK et al. Is there a relationship between leptin and insulin sensitivity independent of obesity? A population-based study in the Indian Ocean nation of Mauritius. *Int J Obes* 1998;22(2):171–177.
40. Wauters M, Considine RV, Gaal LFV. Human leptin: From an adipocyte hormone to an endocrine mediator. *Eur J Endocrinol* 2000;143(3):293–311.
41. Yadav A, Kataria MA, Saini A, Yadav A. Role of leptin and adiponectin in insulin resistance. *Clin Chim Acta* 2013;413:80–84.
42. Dostalova I, Haluzikova D, Haluzik M. Fibroblast growth factor 21: A novel metabolic regulator with potential therapeutic properties in obesity/type 2 diabetes mellitus. *Physiol Res* 2009;58(1):1–7.
43. Zhang J, Yang L. Fibroblast growth factor 21, the endocrine FGF pathway and novel treatments for metabolic syndrome. *Drug Discov Today* 2014;19(5):579–589.
44. Zhang X, Yeung DCY, Karpisek M, Stejskal D, Zhou ZG, Liu F et al. Serum FGF21 levels are increased in obesity and are independently associated With the metabolic syndrome in humans. *Diabetes* 2008;57(5):1246–1253.
45. Fisher FM, Chui PC, Antonellis PJ, Bina HA, Kharitonenkov A, Flier JS. Obesity is a fibroblast growth factor 21 (FGF21)-resistant state. *Diabetes* 2010;59(11):2781–2789.
46. Semba RD, Sun K, Egan JM, Crasto C, Carlson OD, Ferrucci L. Relationship of serum fibroblast growth factor 21 with abnormal glucosemetabolism and insulin resistance: The Baltimore longitudinal study of aging. *J Clin Endocrinol Metab* 2012;97(4):1375–1382.
47. Kralisch S, Tonjes A, Krause K, Richter J, Lossner U, Kovacs P et al. Fibroblast growth factor-21 serum concentrations are associated with metabolic and hepatic markers in humans. *J Endocrinol* 2013;216(2):135–143.
48. Chavez AO, Folli F, Carrion MM, DeFronzo RA, Abdul-Ghani MA, Tripathy D. Circulating fibroblast growth Factor-21 is elevated in impaired glucose tolerance and type 2 diabetes and correlates With muscle and hepatic insulin resistance. *Diabetes Care* 2009;32(8):1542–1546.
49. Storlein LH, Jenkins AB, Chisholm DJ, Pascoe WS, Khouri S, Kraegen EW et al. Influence of dietary fat composition on development of insulin resistance in rats. Relationship to muscle triglyceride and omega-3 fatty acids in muscle phospholipid. *Diabetes* 1991;40(2):280–289.
50. Deer J, Koska J, Ozias M, Reaven P. Dietary models of insulin resistance. *Metabolism* 2015;64(2):163–171.
51. Storlien LH, Kraegen EW, Chisholm DJ, Bruce DG, Pascoe WS. Fish oil prevents insulin resistance induced by high-fat feeding in rats. *Science* 1987;237(4817):885–888.

52. Shulman GI. Cellular mechanisms of insulin resistance. *J Clin Invest* 2000;106(2):171–176.
53. Haag M, Dippenaar NG. Dietary fats, fatty acids and insulin resistance: Short review of a multifaceted connection. *Med Sci Monit* 2005;11(12):RA359–RA367.
54. Sears B, Perry M. The role of fatty acids in insulin resistance. Lipids Health Dis. 2015; 14: 121
55. de Souza RJ, Mente A, Maroleanu A, et al. Intake of saturated and trans unsaturated fatty acids and risk of all cause mortality, cardiovascular disease, and type 2 diabetes: systematic review and meta-analysis of observational studies. BMJ. 2015; 351: h3978.
56. Aune D, Norat T, Romundstad P, Vatten LJ. Dairy products and the risk of type 2 diabetes: a systematic review and dose-response meta-analysis of cohort studies. Am J Clin Nutr. 2013; 98(4): 1066–1083.
57. DiNicolantonio JJ, O'Keefe JH. Importance of maintaining a low omega-6/omega-3 ratio for reducing inflammation. Open Heart. 2018; 5(2): e000946.
58. Maszewska M, Florowska A, Dłużewska E, Wroniak M, Marciniak-Lukasiak K, Żbikowska A. Oxidative Stability of Selected Edible Oils. Molecules. 2018; 23(7): 1746.
59. Awada M, Soulage CO, Meynier A, et al. Dietary oxidized n-3 PUFA induce oxidative stress and inflammation: role of intestinal absorption of 4-HHE and reactivity in intestinal cells. J Lipid Res. 2012; 53(10): 2069–2080.
60. Hwang IS, Ho H, Hoffman BB, Reaven GM. Fructose-induced insulin resistance and hypertension in rats. *Hypertension* 1987;10(5):512–516.
61. Thorburn AW, Storlein LH, Jenkins AB, Khouri S, Kraegen EW. Fructose-induced in vivo insulin resistance and elevated plasma triglyceride levels in rats. *Am J Clin Nutr* 1989;49(6):1155–1163.
62. Basciano H, Federico L, Adeli K. Fructose, insulin resistance, and metabolic dyslipidemia. *Nutr Metab* 2005;2(1):5.

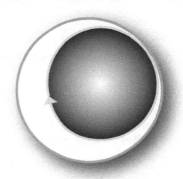

4 Diabetes
A Leading Contributor to Other Disease Complications

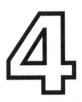

INTRODUCTION

Type 2 diabetes mellitus (T2DM) is currently considered as the most widely diagnosed non-communicable disease in adults around the globe. The reasons behind T2DM extend from genetic predisposition, obesity, sedentary lifestyle, environmental factors, polycystic ovary syndrome (PCOS) and unhealthy dietary habits. The WHO predicted the number of diabetic patients to be approximately 422 million in the year 2014 [1]. The three basic symptoms encountered by T2DM patients are unusual polyuria (frequent urination mainly nocturia), polydipsia (excessive thirst) and polyphagia (excessive hunger). These three basis and other associated symptoms are briefly explained below:

Frequent urination: Excessive thirst and frequent urination are classic symptoms of diabetes. If body insulin is ineffective, or not there at all, the kidneys cannot filter the glucose back into the blood. The kidneys will take water from the blood in order to dilute the glucose – which in turn fills up the bladder.

Disproportionate thirst: If urinating more than usual, the individual will need to replace that lost liquid. The person will be drinking more than usual.

Intense hunger: As the insulin in the blood is not working properly, or is not there at all, and cells are not getting their energy, the body may react by trying to find more energy from food.

Weight gain: This might be the result of the above symptom (intense hunger).

Unusual weight loss: This is more common among people with T1DM. As the body is not making insulin, it will seek out another energy source (the cells are not getting glucose). Muscle tissue and fat will be broken down for energy requirements. As T1DM is of a more sudden onset and T2DM is much more gradual, weight loss is more noticeable with T1DM.

Increased fatigue: If insulin is not working properly, or is not there at all, glucose will not be entering your cells and providing them with energy. This will make the person feel tired and listless.

Irritability: Irritability can be due to your lack of energy.

Blurred vision: This can be caused by tissue being pulled from eye lenses. This affects the eyes' ability to focus. There are severe cases where blindness or prolonged vision problems can occur.

Cuts and bruises don't heal properly or quickly: When there is more sugar (glucose) in the body, its ability to heal can be undermined.

More skin infections: When there is more sugar in your body, its ability to recover from infections is affected. Women with diabetes find it especially difficult to recover from bladder and vaginal infections.

Itchy skin: A feeling of itchiness on the skin is sometimes a symptom of diabetes.

Swollen gums: Gums are red and pull away from teeth. If gums are tender, red and/ or swollen, this could be a sign of diabetes.

Frequent gum disease: As well as the previous gum symptoms, people may experience more frequent gum disease and/or gum infections.

Sexual dysfunction: If persons are over 50 and experience frequent or constant sexual dysfunction, it could be a symptom of diabetes.

Numbness or tingling: If there is too much sugar in the body, nerves could be damaged, as could the tiny blood vessels that feed those nerves. The person may experience tingling and/or numbness in the hands and feet.

Diabetes is mainly diagnosed using HbA1c or plasma glucose measurement such as fasting plasma glucose (FPG), 2-hour post-prandial glucose (PPG) and 75 gram oral glucose tolerance test (OGTT). The criteria for the diagnosis of diabetes using the mentioned parameters are HbA1c ≥ 6.5, FPG ≥ 126 mg/dl (7 mmol/L), PPG ≥ 200 mg/dl (11.1 mmol/L) in the oral glucose tolerance test (OGTT). Among these, HbA1c is considered more appropriate as it reveals the glycaemic condition in the last 3 months [2]. Weight loss is also experienced by patients showing uncontrolled hyperglycaemia. The uncontrolled high blood glucose leads to serious health complications. Diabetes is considered a major risk factor, giving rise to cardiovascular disease and stroke and diabetic patients have a two to four times increased risk of these diseases. Other major pathologies include retinopathy, nephropathy and neuropathy [3].

PATHOPHYSIOLOGY OF T2DM

Our body utilises the glucose obtained from food immediately, or it is converted to glycogen and stored in the liver and muscles as storage polysaccharide or adipose triglyceride (energy reservoir). Insulin is the hormone which controls this action. Diabetes mellitus occurs when the body is no longer capable of taking the blood glucose inside cells and utilise the glucose for different cellular activities. T2DM occurs when the body is either not able to utilise the insulin produced (insulin resistance) or is not producing enough insulin (damage to β-cells due to glucotoxicity). A decreased insulin secretion results from impairment in glucose response by insulin secreting β-cells of the pancreas. A mutation in the glucokinase gene, which plays an important role in the glucose-sensing mechanism of pancreatic beta cells, is also an important factor of impaired glucose tolerance in the pancreas. Insulin resistance, on the other hand, is the condition when the insulin receptors become less responsive towards insulin even when the hormone is present in a physiological amount. This condition is attributed to many factors; the major factor being obesity, which exerts its effect via free fatty acids and inflammatory cytokines (such as TNF-α) which downregulate the insulin receptor and insulin receptor substrate (IRS) protein [4, 5].

DIABETES-RELATED COMPLICATIONS

The American Diabetes Association (ADA) states that a diabetes patient, as compared to a non-diabetic one, has an approximately 7-year shorter life span due to various diabetes-related comorbidities. Some major complications include diabetic retinopathy, neuropathy, coronary artery disease, stroke, peripheral vascular disorders and nephropathy. Diabetic patients are more prone to acquiring cardiovascular complications, cancer and renal failure because of their increased susceptibility towards these diseases [6]. To make it easy for the readers, the two major classification of diabetes comorbidity based on damage to vasculature are microvascular disease (retinopathy, neuropathy and nephropathy) and macrovascular disease (such as cardiovascular disease and peripheral vascular disease). Most of the complications related to diabetes have been attributed to the formation of advanced glycation end-products (AGEs), which are the derivatives of physiological macromolecules. In the case of hyperglycaemia, glucose gets attached to various macromolecules such as proteins in a non-enzymatic reaction, commonly known as the Millard reaction. These new glycated entities lose their normal function and become a health threat, resulting in various complications. The most common example of AGE is glycated haemoglobin or HbA1c which is the most reliable assessment marker to diagnose diabetes and its seriousness [7]. Figure 4.1 shows various comorbidities associated with diabetes.

Diabetic Retinopathy

Diabetic retinopathy (DR) is a result of microvascular damage to the retina due to prolonged hyperglycaemia. DR is mostly irreversible and has become a major cause of

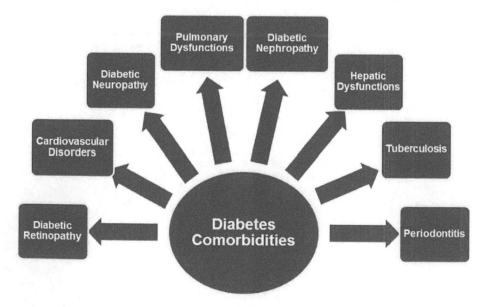

Figure 4.1 Comorbidities associated with diabetes mellitus.

blindness in people with uncontrolled hyperglycaemia. DR is broadly classified into non-proliferative and proliferative forms, based on the progressive clinical stage. During the non-proliferative state, the retinal damage occurs due to abnormal permeability and loss of perfusion of the capillaries which results in the formation of a microaneurysm in the retina. This abnormal permeability further results in leakage of fluids and solutes which finally accumulates around the macula of the eye. This formation of a macular oedema (ME) poses a threat to the vision. When retinal capillaries get occluded, they lead to a condition called retinal ischaemia. Neovascularisation (formation of new blood vessels) follows the retinal ischaemia. Since the new blood vessels have less integrity and are fragile, they result in haemorrhage. The resulting accumulation of leaked blood becomes a serious threat to vision. According to estimates, 50% of the diabetic population with DR will become blind without treatment within 5 years of initial diagnosis [8]. The disease occurs due to alteration in retinal vasculature and damage to ocular nerves. The Diabetes Research Centre (India) conducted a study on 1,000 diabetic patients which revealed that retinopathy increased linearly with progressing diabetes [9]. The Madras Diabetes Research Foundation (India) conducted another study which revealed that diabetic retinopathy is associated with increased thickness of intima-media and stiffness of ocular vessels and that DR starts developing years before the diagnosis of diabetes is made if there is uncontrolled hyperglycaemia for 3–4 years [10]. Comparing the occurrence of DR in Indian and Western populations, keeping the age, gender and duration of the disease the same, it was found that while the south Indian population had a DR percentage of 17.6, it was around 30 for the Western population [11].

Glutamate, which is an excitatory neurotransmitter, gets transported to synaptic vesicles by VGLUT1 (glutamate vesicular transporter 1) which is the major transporter expressed in photoreceptors. A study has shown that VGLUT1 expression decreases in the retina of diabetic mice and was not normalised even after treatment with metformin [12]. A recent finding shows that the expression of the enzyme phospholipase A_2 (PLA_2) is upregulated early in glucose-induced alteration of the retinal layer. The expression level of PLA_2, COX-2 and VEGF were found to be significantly increased in retinal microvessels of the diabetic rat model [13]. Retinal pericytes maintain a microvascular homeostasis but they gradually accumulate AGEs in the case of prolonged hyperglycaemia, which results in endothelial dysfunction. It has also been viewed that the accumulated AGEs activate NF-κB which increases the oxidative stress in pericytes and other retinal cells with increased production of reactive oxygen species (ROS) which results in increased apoptosis [14]. The polyol pathway is another important biochemical pathological implication of prolonged hyperglycaemia which is a key risk factor of DR. Retinal cells are insulin-independent cells and thus glucose can freely move inside. Glucose is converted to sorbitol and then to fructose, using the polyol pathway. The two enzymes in this pathway are aldose reductase (AR) and sorbitol dehydrogenase. AR is considered as the rate limiting enzyme of the polyol pathway. Since AR has low affinity towards glucose, in the case of normoglycaemia, much less glucose gets converted to sorbitol by AR. During the hyperglycaemic state, excess glucose is converted to sorbitol in large amounts. This reaction utilises excess NADPH; therefore, a reduction in NADPH, in turn, leads to a reduced amount of glutathione and increased oxidative stress. This increased oxidative stress is a great contributor to retinal damage [15]. Other important pathological alterations due to hyperglycaemia that pose great risks for DR development are increased expression of poly (ADP-ribose) polymerase (PARP), increased hexosamine content of the retina and protein kinase C enzyme (PKC) which again increases the oxidative stress of the retinal cells [14, 15].

Cardiovascular Disorders

Cardiovascular disorders are one of the most notorious complications arising from uncontrolled diabetes. Uncontrolled prolonged hyperglycaemia results in the formation of AGEs (glycation products) on the physiological proteins and lipids which disrupts their normal functions and results in various pathological conditions. RAGEs (immunoglobulin superfamily), which are the receptors for AGE, have an influential effect on the physiological cellular signalling upon binding with AGEs. Cross-linking of AGEs with elastin protein and type I collagen in endothelial walls results in stiffness of vasculature. Various studies suggest that glycated lipids such as glycated LDL reduces the nitric oxide (NO) production in endothelium and suppresses LDL receptor mediated LDL uptake by endothelial cells. Physiologically, NO is one of the most potent natural vasodilators. AGE-induced suppression of NO production from endothelial cells in diabetic patients is considered an important factor resulting in arteriosclerosis and atherosclerosis as nitric oxide exhibits a wide range of anti-atherogenic actions, such as inhibition of platelet adhesion and aggregation, inhibition of leukocyte adhesion to endothelial walls of blood vessel, etc. [16, 17]. A range of cardiovascular complications, such as stroke, myocardial infarction and cardiac failure, are the result of AGE-induced arterial stiffness and platelets adhesion and aggregation that can lead to overall mortality. Myocardial stiffness due to cross-linking of glycated extracellular matrix (ECM) collagen in myocardium leads to left ventricular hypertrophy (LVH) which in turn causes pressure overload. The suppression of LDL receptor mediated LDL uptake can pose a significant risk of atherosclerosis leading to occlusion in blood flow in major coronary arteries. The pathological symptoms start with (in progressive order) hypertension, ischaemia, infarction and finally cardiac attack. Unregulated prolonged diabetes, therefore, can be seen as a critical risk factor towards cardiovascular disorders [18–20].

The Madras Diabetes Research Foundation (India) and Indian Diabetes Research Foundation (India) independently conducted various studies in India and concluded that Indians, especially the south Indian population, are at high risk of developing diabetes, insulin resistance and related cardiovascular complications. The primary risk factors observed in these studies, involving wide age group subjects, were low level of high-density lipoprotein (low HDL) and high triglyceride (TG) level, contributing to an increased risk of metabolic syndrome [21–23]. Diabetic cardiomyopathy can be defined as myocardial dysfunction in diabetic patients in the absence of coronary artery disease (CAD), hypertension and valve defects. The development of diabetic cardiomyopathy is attributed to various factors viz. insulin resistance, hyperlipidaemia and cardiac autonomic dysfunction. Insulin resistance and hyperlipidaemia are two major ingredients of a collective complication known as metabolic syndrome (MS). Hyperglycaemia, hyperinsulinaemia and elevated free fatty acid (FFA) are the major factors that lead to cardiac steatosis. Brain natriuretic peptide (BNP), biomolecule released from cardiac ventricles, was also found to be elevated in patients who suffered heart failure. The gene expression of BNP was also found to be upregulated in animal models of insulin resistance (hyperinsulinaemia) along with other symptoms such as LVH [24].

Diabetic Nephropathy

Renal disorder is another major diabetic comorbidity. Prolonged hyperglycaemia results in glomerulosclerosis which increases thickness of the basement membrane and further causes microaneurysm, hyaline arteriosclerosis and diffused mesangial sclerosis with nodule formation. This chain of renal pathologies eventually results in microalbuminuria, followed by macroalbuminuria, proceeding to the loss of the glomerular filtration rate (GFR) and probable end stage renal disease (ESRD). A study conducted on diabetic patients in the United States demonstrated that the patients had increased albuminuria (albumin in urine) and high systolic pressure as compared to non-diabetic subjects. It is estimated that almost half of the patients with renal disorder having renal replacement therapy in the United States suffer from T2DM [25]. According to an Indian study conducted between 2009 and 2011, it was demonstrated that microalbuminuria was elevated in the population with uncontrolled hyperglycaemia which led to an increased level of serum creatinine which is indicative of renal damage with high significance (p<0.0001) [26]. Persistent and prolonged proteinuria and albuminuria also result in renal tubule dysfunction which is attributed to damage of the epithelial layer due to continuous flow of plasma protein. This results in a condition known as tubulointerstitial fibrosis which leads to irreversible renal damage. Serum cystatin C (Cys C; 13 kD protein), a low molecular weight non-glycosylated proteinase, is known to be completely filtered through glomerulus and almost completely catabolised by the tubular epithelium [27]. It was demonstrated by a recent study conducted on 70 diabetic and 20 control subjects that the serum Cys C level was significantly elevated in diabetic patients compared to the age, weight and gender equated control subjects, and it also has a positively correlation with urine albumin and creatinine secretion [28]. At the molecular level, diabetic nephropathy is also characterised by excessive deposition of the extra-cellular matrix (ECM) proteins in the mesangial cells of the basement membrane and renal tubulointerstitium attributed to increased oxidative stress (ROS generation) and upregulation of TGF-β, with a decreased expression of matrix metalloproteinases (MMP). This is followed by an increase in glomerular basement membrane thickness. Other pathophysiological changes include significant glomerulosclerosis [29]. A recent article reviewed extensively various biomarkers related to renal damage. Neutrophil gelatinase associated lipocalin (NGAL), which is a 25 kD protein, has come up as a sensitive biomarker in the case of diabetic nephropathy. Appearance of NGAL in urine is considered as an early marker of renal injury as it appears much earlier than albumin. It was found to be significantly higher in diabetic patients than non-diabetic subjects. Urine NGAL was positively correlated to serum Cys C, creatinine and serum urea, while inversely correlated to GFR. N-acetyl-beta-glucosaminidase (NAG) is an enzyme produced in the lysosome of epithelial cells of proximal tubules. Its appearance in urine is a very early indicator of renal damage. It was even found to be elevated in T2D patients with normoalbuminuria. NAG was demonstrated to have higher sensitivity than serum creatinine, and therefore, it is treated as a better early marker of diabetic nephropathy. Alpha-1 microglobulin (A1MG), type IV collagen, nephrin and angiotensinogen are other very sensitive biomarkers that are indicative of very early renal damage [30].

Diabetic Neuropathy

Diabetic peripheral neuropathy (DPN) is one of the major complications of uncontrolled hyperglycaemia affecting approximately 50% of type 2 diabetes patients who do not receive proper diagnosis and treatment. DPN is broadly defined as distal, symmetric and sensorimotor neuropathy. Approximately 30% of diabetes patients exhibit painful neuropathy, while the remainder experience numbness and loss of sensation. The disease is clinically determined by poor gait pattern and balance (associated with large sensory fibres) and abnormal heat and cold sensation (associated with small sensory fibres). Among all neuropathic conditions associated with diabetes, distal symmetric polyneuropathy (DSP) is the most common. It is said that diabetic patients with DSP have two to three times more chance of falling due to loss of balance compared to a diabetic patient without DSP. Other types of neuropathy that can affect patients with diabetes are small fibre predominant neuropathy, radiculoplexopathy, mononeuritis multiplex and autonomic neuropathy. Autonomic neuropathy, which is also common with prolonged hyperglycaemia, displays symptoms such as gastroparesis, constipation, erectile dysfunction, urinary retention and cardiac arrhythmias. It is important to note that autonomic neuropathy can severely destroy quality of life and can even be fatal [31]. DPN patients often complain of chronic pain and common symptoms such as itching, tingling and 'pins and needles poking sensation', bee sting, etc. The chronic pain experienced by some patients can be described as allodynia (pain from normal stimuli), hyperesthesias (increased sensitivity to touch) and hyperalgesia (increased sensitivity to painful stimuli). The advanced stage of DPN affects the limbs and commonly leads to diabetic foot (ulceration in the affected lower limb). Diabetic neuropathic pain, as described by the International Association for the Study of Pain, is 'a pain arising as a direct consequence of abnormalities in peripheral somatosensory system in people with diabetes' [32]. A recent study conducted on DPN patients and control subjects has shown a positive correlation between serum TNF-α and DPN [33].

Diabetic foot infection (DFI) is often the most common and disturbing result of peripheral neuropathy that begins with a neuropathic ulceration in the affected limb. Vascular insufficiency and diminished neutrophil function further enhance the DPN which results in infection. DFIs are primarily associated with aerobic gram-positive cocci, especially staphylococci, and aerobic gram-negative bacilli as the causative co-pathogens [34]. The most common organisms colonising the infected area are beta-haemolysing streptococci and *Staphylococcus aureus*. Apart from these microorganisms, *Klebsiella*, *E. coli* and methicillin-resistant Staphylococcus aureus (MRSA) are common inhabitants, resulting in severely debilitating infections [35].

Pulmonary Dysfunctions

Pulmonary disorders are perhaps the most neglected comorbidity in diabetic patients. Most commonly, glycated collagen has been observed to be deposited in the lung parenchyma and chest walls, which in turn increases the stiffness of lungs, leading to a reduction in their expansion. The neuropathic changes also affect the respiratory muscles. Obesity, which is a major contributor to T2D, has been related to increased leptin level insulin resistance. Obese-diabetic patients significantly develop chronic ailments such as obstructive asthma, sleep apnoea, chronic obstructive pulmonary disorder (COPD) and lung cancer. It is also described that diabetic patients have reduced pulmonary diffusing capacity for carbon monoxide (DLCO) due to vascular injury to capillaries in the lungs due to microangiopathy. The pulmonary system is extremely susceptible to non-enzymatic glycation and related microvascular damage due to extensive vascularity. The organ is particularly very susceptible to protein glycation due to its richness in elastin and collagen [36]. It has been reported that prolonged uncontrolled hyperglycaemia results in lower forced expiratory volume in 1 second (FEV1) and forced vital capacity (FVC) in diabetic patients as compared to normal subjects [37]. The effect of AGEs is so intense that the histopathological examination of the lungs of diabetic patients has clear evidence of thickened epithelial, alveolar and capillary basal lamina. Hyperglycaemia also leads to pulmonary vascular damage that leads to diabetic microangiopathy [38]. A strong positive correlation was found between hyperglycaemia and deteriorating lung function with a reduction in FEV and FVC in an Indian study involving 40 diabetic patients [39]. Volumes of basal laminae, extracellular matrix and interstitial connective tissue are increased in lungs of streptozotocin-induced type 1 diabetic rats as compared to the control group. Alveolar type 2 epithelial cells were also altered in morphology. This experimentally induced T1DM was also associated with increased triglyceride deposits and diminished phospholipid content of the lungs.

The expression of surfactant protein SP-A and SP-B was also significantly reduced in the experimental animal models, but was normal in the control group [40]. Babies delivered to diabetic mothers are at an increased risk of pulmonary dysfunctions such as intrauterine or perinatal asphyxia. The foetus also develops the above condition when the mother has vascular dysfunctions due to diabetes. Moreover, respiratory distress syndrome (RDS) occurs more frequently in infants born to diabetic mothers than to non-diabetic mothers, mostly when delivery is done <38.5 weeks. This is possibly because hyperinsulinaemia diminishes the surfactant maturity. Transient tachypnoea of the newborn (TTN) is also seen almost two to three times more often in infants born to diabetic mothers than in those born to non-diabetic mothers [41]. A recent study involving computed tomography (CT) scans of diabetic and control groups revealed that the permeability surface of lungs was significantly higher in diabetic patients compared to the non-diabetic control group due to diabetes induced microangiopathy. There was a significant difference in vital capacity and total lung capacity between the two groups [42]. Autonomic neuropathy of lungs, in diabetes, results in depressed cholinergic bronchomotor tone and neuroadrenergic denervation. It was found that almost 30% of patients with uncontrolled hyperglycaemia displayed abnormal ventilator response to hypercapnia and hypoxia. Increased permeability to macromolecules due to increased vascular permeability followed by intense accumulation of caveolae and overexpression of endothelial caveolin-1 results in increased thickness of alveolar epithelium and endothelial diffusion barrier in diabetic patients [43].

Hepatic Dysfunction

T2D is an important risk factor for the development of non-alcohol fatty liver disease (NAFLD) and other chronic liver diseases. Non-alcoholic steatohepatitis (NASH), a chronic necro-inflammatory condition, is probably the most severe form of NAFLD that results in fibrosis, cirrhosis and finally hepatocellular carcinoma (HCC). In a large cohort study published almost a decade ago, it was found that T2DM doubled the risk of NAFLD and HCC. One important mechanism underlying this pathological change is increased peripheral lipolysis due to insulin resistance leading to accumulation of free fatty acids (FFA) in the liver, resulting in NAFLD. The hepatic damage is attributed to cellular necrosis and inflammation which occurs due to increased mitochondrial oxidative stress. Further damage is conceived by increased production of inflammatory cytokines such as TNF-α. The hepatic damage further worsens the diabetic state as the liver is the prime site of carbohydrate metabolism and insulin action. The secondary diabetes which occurs due to this hepatic damage is known as hepatogenous diabetes [44, 45]. Another human cohort study conducted between 1994 and 2006 revealed that diabetic patients had higher risk of developing serious hepatic dysfunctional pathology compared to the non-diabetic control subjects [46]. Another large human study involving over 1.7 lakhs diabetic patients and 6.5 lakhs non-diabetic control subjects revealed that diabetes increases the risk of acute hepatic failure by almost one-and-a-half times [47]. A large meta-analysis revealed the liver enzyme alanine transaminase (ALT) was commonly elevated in T2DM patients, while uncommon in normal subjects. Patients with T2DM had higher incidence of liver cirrhosis, acute hepatic failure, hepatocellular carcinoma and they were at higher risk of hepatitis C [48].

OTHER COMPLICATIONS

Periodontitis

Periodontitis is considered an important consequence of uncontrolled diabetes. The National Health and Nutrition Examination Survey and the Hispanic Health and Nutrition Survey, based on US epidemiological data, revealed that the diabetic population has high prevalence of periodontal pockets as compared to the non-diabetic control group. It was also reported that T2DM increased the risk of periodontitis by three times. The gingival membrane and capillaries of the diabetic patients were found to be considerably dysfunctional than those in the non-diabetic control group. Apart from these gingival vascular changes, other sub-gingival changes have also been reported in diabetes. Upon the induction of diabetes in rats, the sub-gingival flora acquired mostly gram-negative bacteria and the periodontal pockets deepened [49]. Mashimo et al. reported that the periodontal lesions in T1DM patients predominantly consisted of *Capnocytophaga* sp. while *Actinobacillus actinomycetemcomitans* was found to be in the cultured sample of periodontitis in three out of nine diabetics [50]. Zambon et al. found that *P. intermedia*, *P. gingivalis* and *W. recta* were the three most prominent pathogens found in the sub-gingival dental plaques of T2DM patients [51]. On the genetic note, patients with type 1 diabetes have a higher predisposition for HLA-DR4. On examining non-diabetic patients with periodontitis, it was found that almost 80% were positive for HLA-DR4 as compared to only 38% in the control population. This revealed that HLA-DR4 predisposed patients have a higher risk of progressive periodontitis [49].

Genito-Urinary Infections

T2D has been a well-known risk factor for balanitis in males and vulvovaginitis in females, which are the most common urinary tract infections (UTI) reported in these genders, respectively. Hyperglycaemia and glycosuria in T2DM favours the growth of *Candida albicans* at the vaginal epithelium because hyperglycaemia is said to interfere with normal host-defence mechanism and aids in the growth of the pathogenic *Candida* sp. [52]. A study conducted in the UK using the General Practice Research Database (GPRD) revealed that T2DM increases the risk of UTI by 60% compared to that in non-diabetic people. T2D also seems to increase the risk of vulvovaginitis two-fold and balanitis three-fold [53].

Tuberculosis

According to an estimate published in an article in 2011, over 2 billion people globally have been infected with *Mycobacterium tuberculosis*, out of which 11 million had active tuberculosis (TB). An epidemiological study in India reported that diabetes accounted for approximately 14.8% of pulmonary TB and 20.2% smear-positive TB. Another point observed in this article is that diabetic patients are supposed to be around five times more susceptible to multi-drug-resistant TB (MDR-TB) [54]. A recent large population-based cohort study (approximately 1.3 lakhs female and 1.3 lakhs male patients) conducted in Taiwan reported that T2DM significantly increased the risk of development of pulmonary tuberculosis (TB). Diabetic patients also had the increased risk of relapse of the disease after successful completion of treatment for TB. They also exhibited high bacillary load in sputum [55]. Diabetes patients are reported to have a lower number of circulating neutrophils and activated macrophages and there is a negative correlation between the elevated HbA1c and phagocytic activity in the macrophages. The phagocytic activity improved significantly when the glucose level came down to normal [56]. In a large meta-analysis of available literatures and studies on the association of T2DM and TB, it was reported that diabetes increases the risk of developing active TB three-fold. The study reported that this increased risk of TB in diabetic subjects persists regardless of study region, background incidence or any other medical condition. The study also observed that diabetic mice infected with *M. tuberculosis* had higher bacterial load as compared to that in the euglycaemic population. The diabetic mice had significantly low levels of IFN-γ, IL-12 and Th1 responsiveness towards mycobacterium which play a crucial role in controlling TB. In the human population too, the state of hyperinsulinaemia resulted in a decrease of Th1 cell and gross reduction in essential protective cytokines. The study also observed that there is a negative correlation between the level of HbA1c and IFN-γ [57].

Gastroparesis

In 1958, Kassender coined the term 'gastroparesis diabeticorum' for the symptom of delayed gastric emptying in diabetic patients. Gastroparesis is a pathological condition where there is delayed gastric emptying without any mechanical or pharmacological inhibition. The classical symptoms of gastroparesis are a sense of early fullness during eating (early satiety), feeling of fullness even long after having a meal which is often accompanied by bloating, nausea and vomiting. Diabetes is considered as one of the major causes with almost one-third of gastroparesis patients being diabetic. Other causes could be gastrointestinal surgery or a neurological problem. Gastroparesis is a chronic complication of diabetes and mostly, such gastroparetic patients also have other diabetes-related complications such as retinopathy and neuropathy. Diabetic patients show gastroparesis primarily due to neuropathy that affects the vagus nerve, and reduction in the number of gastric pacemaker cells (interstitial cells of Cajal or ICC). This neuropathy complication is a part of a larger neuropathy conglomeration known as diabetic autonomic neuropathy (DAN). The gastroparetic symptoms can become worse in diabetic patients taking certain medications such as amylin analogue (Pramlintide) or GLP-1 analogues (e.g. Exenatide). Specifically, diabetes-related gastric symptoms could be divided into oesophageal dysmotility, gastroparesis and diabetic enteropathies (intestinal dysmotility, diarrhoea and faecal incontinence). The American College of Gastroenterology (ACG) suggests that a combination of suitable symptoms along with delayed gastric emptying without any mechanical or pharmacological interventions is essential to diagnose diabetic gastroparesis [58, 59]. The techniques which are commonly applied to diagnose diabetic gastroparesis are gastric scintigraphy, ultrasonography, magnetic resonance imaging (MRI), single-photon emission computed tomography, electrogastrography (EGG) and wireless motility capsule (smart pill). While the management of gastroparesis includes diet and lifestyle management, diabetic patients suffering from gastroparesis must manage their diabetes through pharmacological treatment as suggested by a physician. Apart from these interventions, certain common medicines used to manage diabetic gastroparesis are Metoclopramide, Domperidone, Erythromycin, Cisapride, phenothiazines, serotonin (5-HT$_3$) receptor antagonists [58, 59].Table 4.1 shows various diabetes-related comorbidities, their pathological markers and the related pathology.

Table 4.1 Diabetes-Related Comorbidities, Markers and Related Pathology

Diabetes-related Comorbidities	Diagnostic Markers	Related Pathology	References
Diabetic retinopathy	Increased PLA2, VEGF, COX-2, Macular oedema, Retinal exudate	Ocular arterial stiffness, Permanent blindness	[8–15]
Cardiovascular disorders	Hypertriglyceridaemia, Hypercholesterolaemia, Circulating RAGE	Arterial stiffness, Atherosclerosis, LVH, Hypertension, etc.	[16–24]
Diabetic nephropathy	High glycated albumin, Increased serum cystatin C, High serum creatinine, Low GFR	Glomerulosclerosis, End stage renal disease	[25–30]
Diabetic neuropathy	Reduction in serum TNF-α	Pain, Numbness, Hyperesthesia, Allodynia, Hyperalgesia, Severe lower limb infections	[31–35]
Pulmonary defects	Reduction in PFTs, elasticity, Parenchymal aberrations	COPD, Obstructive sleep apnoea, Lung cancer	[36–43]
Hepatic dysfunction	Lipid accumulation in hepatocytes, Elevated liver enzymes	NAFLD, Cirrhosis, HCC	[44–48]
Periodontitis	Damage in gingival membrane and vasculature, Pathogenic microbial colonisation	Periodontal pocket formation, Infection	[49–51]
Genito-urinary infections	Infection diagnosis by various means (no specific biomarker)	Primarily candidiasis	[52–53]
Tuberculosis	Lower circulating neutrophils and macrophages, Low IFN-γ, IL-12	Pulmonary tuberculosis, MDR-TB	[54–57]
Gastroparesis	Delayed gastric emptying, Bloating, Nausea (no biomarker available)	Gastrointestinal pathologies	[58, 59]

CONCLUSIONS

Diabetes is considered as the most widely propagating non-communicable disease which is gradually becoming an epidemic. Diabetic patients are shown to be affected by an array of pathologies such as neuropathy, cardiovascular diseases, retinopathy, pulmonary dysfunctions, etc. Diabetic retinopathy is gradually becoming the biggest cause of blindness across the globe. Uncontrolled hyperglycaemia is surely going to result in a cardiac problem at some stage in life. Organ dysfunction, which is avoidable by good control over hyperglycaemia, significantly affects quality of life and has been the major reason for diabetic comorbidity. Diabetic patients are also susceptible to various infections which respond poorly to the available antibiotic treatments. Even serious communicable diseases such as TB have a significantly greater chance of occurrence in patients with diabetes. The WHO prediction on the number of diabetic patients has become a challenge globally. Following a healthy lifestyle can result in a significant reduction in the incidence of diabetes, which is a non-expensive method that can be easily followed.

REFERENCES

1. WHO. Global report on Diabetes 2016. Accessed at http://apps.who.int/iris/bitst ream/10665/204871/1/9789241565257_eng.pdf?ua=1&ua=1; accessed on May 25, 2018.
2. American diabetes association classification and diagnosis of diabetes: Standards of medical care in diabetes-2018. *Diabetes Care* 2018;41(Suppl 1):S13–S27.
3. Accessed at www.who.int/diabetes/action_online/basics/en/index1.html; accessed on May 25, 2018.
4. Taylor SI. Deconstructing Type 2 diabetes. *Cell* 1999;97(1):9–12.
5. Kaku K. Pathophysiology of Type 2 diabetes and its treatment policy. *J Jpn Med Assoc* 2010;53(1):41–46.
6. American Diabetes Association. Standards of medical care in diabetes-2013. *Diabetes Care* 2013;36(1):S11–S66.
7. Ottum MS, Mistry AM. Advanced glycation end-products: Modifiable environmental factors profoundly mediate insulin resistance. *J Clin Biochem Nutr* 2015;57(1):1–12.
8. Williams R, Airey M, Baxter H, Forrester H, Martin TK, Girach A. Epidemiology of diabetic retinopathy and macular oedema: A systematic review. *Eye* 2004;18(10):963–983.
9. Ramachandran A, Snehalatha C, Vijay V, Viswanathan M. Diabetic retinopathy at the time of diagnosis of T2DM in south Indian subjects. *Diabetes Res Clin Pract* 1996;32(1–2):111–114.
10. Rema M, Pradeepa R. Diabetic retinopathy: An Indian perspective. *Indian J Med Res* 2007;125(3):297–310.
11. Unnikrishnan R, Anjana RM, Mohan V. Diabetes mellitus and its complications in India. *Nat Rev Endocrinol* 2016;12(6):357–370.
12. Ly A, Scheerer MF, Zukunft S, Muschet C, Merl J, Adamski J et al. Retinal proteome alterations in a mouse model of type 2 diabetes. *Diabetologia* 2014;57(1):192–203.
13. Lupo G, Motta C, Giurdanella G, Anfuso CD, Alberghina M, Drago F et al. Role of phospholipases A2 in diabetic retinopathy: In vitro and in vivo studies. *Biochem Pharmacol* 2013;13:00580–00587.

14. Ola MS, Nawaz MI, Siddiquei MM, Al-Amro A, El-Asrar AMA. Recent advances in understanding the biochemical and molecular mechanism of diabetic retinopathy. *J Diabetes Complications* 2012;26(1):56–64.
15. Brownlee M. Biochemistry and molecular cell biology of diabetic complications. *Nature* 2001;414(6865):813–820.
16. Murea M, Ma L, Freedman BI. Genetic and environmental factors associated with type 2 diabetes and diabetic vascular complications. Rev Diab Std 2012;9(1):6–22.
17. Goldin A, Beckman JA, Schmidt AM. Advanced glycation end products: Sparking the development of diabetic vascular injury. *Circulation* 2006;114(6):597–605.
18. Zieman S, Kass D. Advanced glycation end product cross-linking: Pathophysiologic role and therapeutic target in cardiovascular disease. *Congest Heart Fail* 2004;10(3):144–151.
19. Barlovic DP, Paavonen AS, Jandeleit-Dahm KAM. RAGE biology, atherosclerosis and diabetes. *Clin Sci (Lond)* 2011;121(2):43–55.
20. Selvin E, Halushka MK, Rawlings AM, Hoogeveen RC, Ballantyne CM, Coresh J et al. sRAGE and risk of diabetes, cardiovascular disease, and death. *Diabetes* 2013;62(6):2116–2121.
21. Mohan V, Sandeep S, Deepa M, Gokulakrishnan K, Datta M, Deepa R. A diabetes risk score helps identify metabolic syndrome and cardiovascular risk in Indians - The Chennai Urban Rural Epidemiology Study (CURES-38). *Diabetes Obes Metab* 2007;9(3):337–343.
22. Sandeep S, Gokulakrishnan K, Deepa M, Mohan V. Insulin resistance is associated with increased cardiovascular risk in Asian Indians with normal glucose tolerance--The Chennai Urban Rural Epidemiology Study (CURES-66). *J Assoc Phys India* 2011;59:480–484.
23. Ramachandran A, Snehalatha C, Yamuna A, Murugesan N, Narayan KM. Insulin resistance and clustering of cardiometabolic risk factors in urban teenagers in Southern India. *Diabetes Care* 2007;30(7):1828–1833.
24. Pappachan JM, Varughese GI, Sriraman R, Arunagirinathan G. Diabetic cardiomyopathy: Pathophysiology, diagnostic evaluation and management. *World J Diabetes* 2013;4(5):177–189.
25. Kramer HJ, Nguyen QD, Curhan G, Hsu CY. Renal insufficiency in absence of albuminuria and retinopathy among adults with type 2 diabetes mellitus. *JAMA* 2003;289(24):3273–3277.
26. Kondaveeti SBDK, Mishra S, Kumar RA, Shaker IA. Evaluation of glycated albumin and microalbuminuria as early risk markers of nephropathy in type 2 diabetes mellitus. *J Clin Diagn Res* 2013;7(7):1280–1283.
27. Dharnidharka VR, Kwon C, Stevens G. Serum cystatin C is superior to serum creatinine as a marker of kidney function: A meta-analysis. *Am J Kidney Dis* 2002;40(2):221–226.
28. Assal HS, Tawfeek S, Rasheed EA, El-Lebedy D, Thabet EH. Serum cystatin C and tubular urinary enzymes as biomarkers of renal dysfunction in type 2 diabetes mellitus. *Clin Med Insights Endocrinol Diabetes* 2013;6:7–13.
29. Mason RM, Wahab NA. Extracellular matrix metabolism in diabetic nephropathy. *J Am Soc Nephrol* 2003;14(5):1358–1373.
30. Fiseha T. Urinary biomarkers for early diabetic nephropathy in type 2 diabetic patients. *Biomark Res* 2015;3:16.
31. Callaghan BC, Cheng H, Stables CL, Smith AL, Feldman EL. Diabetic neuropathy: Clinical manifestations and current treatments. *Lancet Neurol* 2012;11(6):521–534.
32. Farmer KL, Li C, Dobrowsky RT. Diabetic peripheral neuropathy: Should a chaperone accompany our therapeutic approach? *Pharmacol Rev* 2012;64(4):880–900.

33. Hussain G, Rizvi SA, Singhal S, Zubair M, Ahmad J. Serum levels of TNF-α in peripheral neuropathy patients and its correlation with nerve conduction velocity in type 2 diabetes mellitus. *Diabetes Metab Syndr* 2013;7(4):238–242.
34. Lipsky BA, Berendt AR, Cornia PB, Pile JC, Peters EJ, Armstrong DG et al. 2012 Infectious Diseases Society of America clinical practice guideline for the diagnosis and treatment of diabetic foot infections. *Clin Infec Dis* 2012;54(12):132–173.
35. Bader MS. Diabetic foot infection. *Am Fam Phys* 2008;78(1):71–79.
36. Pitocco D, Fuso L, Conte EG, Zaccardi F, Condoluci C, Scavone G et al. The diabetic lung - A new target organ? *Rev Diabet Stud* 2012;9(1):23–35.
37. Dharwadkar AR, Dharwadkar AA, Banu G, Bagali S. Reduction in lung functions in type-2 diabetes in Indian population: Correlation with glycemic status. *Indian J Physiol Pharmacol* 2011;55(2):170–175.
38. Aparna A. Pulmonary function tests in type 2 diabetics and non-diabetic people -A comparative study. *J Clin Diagn Res* 2013;7(8):1606–1608.
39. Shah SH, Sonawane P, Nahar P, Vaidya S, Salvi S. Pulmonary function tests in type 2 diabetes mellitus and their association with glycemic control and duration of the disease. *Lung India* 2013;30(2):108–112.
40. Foster DJ, Ravikumar P, Bellotto DJ, Unger RH, Hsia CCW. Fatty diabetic lung: Altered alveolar structure and surfactant protein expression. *Am J Physiol Lung Cell Mol Physiol* 2010;298(3):L392–L403.
41. Milla CE, Zirbes J. Pulmonary complications of endocrine and metabolic disorders. *Paed Resp Rev* 2012;13(1):23–28.
42. Kuziemski K, Pien'kowska J, Słomin'ski W, Jassem E, Studniarek M. Pulmonary Capillary permeability and pulmonary microangiopathy in diabetes mellitus. *Diab Res Clin Pract* 2015;108:e56–e59.
43. Hsia CCW, Raskin P. Lung function changes related to diabetes mellitus. *Diabetes Technol Ther* 2007;9(1):S73–S82.
44. El-Serag HB, Tran T, Everhart JE. Diabetes increases the risk of chronic liver disease and hepatocellular carcinoma. *Gastroenterology* 2004;126(2):460–468.
45. Compean DG, Quintana JOJ, Gonzalez JAG, Garza HM. Liver cirrhosis and diabetes: Risk factors, pathophysiology, clinical implications and management. *World J Gastroenterol* 2009;15(3):280–288.
46. Porepa L, Ray JG, Romeu PS, Booth GL. Newly diagnosed diabetes mellitus as a risk factor for serious liver disease. *Can Med Ass J* 2010;182(11):E526–E531.
47. El-Serag HB, Everhart JE. Diabetes increases the risk of acute hepatic failure. *Gastroenterology* 2002;122(7):1822–1828.
48. Tolman KG, Dalpiaz A, Fonseca V, Tan MH. Spectrum of liver disease in Type 2 diabetes and management of patients with diabetes and liver disease. *Diabetes Care* 2007;30(3):734–743.
49. Oliver RC, Tervonen T. Diabetes—A risk factor for periodontitis in adults? *J Periodontol* 1994;65(5):530–538.
50. Mashimo PA, Yamamoto Y, Slots J, Park BH, Genco RJ. The periodontal microflora of juvenile diabetics. Culture, immunoflourescence and serum antibody studies. *J Periodontal* 1983;54(7):420–430.
51. Zambón JJ, Reynolds H, Fisher JG, Schlossman M, Dunford R, Genco R. Microbiological and immunological studies of adult Periodontitis in patients with non-insulin dependent diabetes mellitus. *J Periodontol* 1988;59(1):23–31.
52. Johnsson KM, Ptaszynska A, Schmitz B, Sugg J, Parikh SJ, List JF. Vulvovaginitis and balanitis in patients with diabetes treated with dapagliflozin. *J Diabetes Complications* 2013;27(5):479–484.

53. Hirji I, Guo Z, Andersson SW, Hammar N, Gomez-Caminero A. Incidence of urinary tract infection among patients with type 2 diabetes in the Uk General Practice Research Database (GPRD). *J Diabetes Complications* 2012;26(6):513–516.
54. Bailey SL, Grant P. 'The tubercular diabetic': The impact of diabetes mellitus on tuberculosis and its threat to global tuberculosis control. *Clin Med (Lond)* 2011;11(4):344–347.
55. Kuo M-C, Lin S-H, Lin C-H, Mao I-C, Chang S-J, Hsieh MC. Type 2 diabetes: An independent risk factor for tuberculosis: A nationwide population based study. *PLoS One* 2013;8(11):e78924.
56. Jepsen DF. The double burden. *Dan Med J* 2013;60(7):B4673.
57. Jeon CY, Murray MB. Diabetes mellitus increases the risk of active tuberculosis: A systematic review of 13 observational studies. *PLoS Med* 2008;5(7):e152.
58. Krishnasamy S, Abell TL. Diabetic gastroparesis: Principles and current Trendsin management. *Diabetes Ther* 2018;9(S1):S1–S42.
59. Camilleri M. Clinical practice: Diabetic gastroparesis. *N Engl J Med* 2007;356(8):820–829.

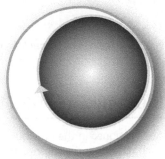

5 Biomarkers of Diabetes

BIOMARKERS

A biomarker is classically defined as any signature molecule, compound, substance or process, or any product thereof, that can be measured in the body to predict the incidence or outcome of a pathological state. Biomarkers play an integral part in conducting clinical trials and treating patients. In most instances, they help medical practitioners, researchers and regulatory officials make well-informed and scientifically relevant decisions. For a disease like T1DM that can initiate at a juvenile age, any biomarker related to that must predict a quantifiable risk and the current disease state too. The major studied biomarkers in T1DM are primarily the serum autoantibodies against the β-cells viz. islet cell antibodies (ICAs), insulin-autoantibodies (IAA), glutamic acid decarboxylase antibodies (GAD-65 autoantibody or GADA), insulinoma-associated antigen-2 autoantibodies (IA-2A) and zinc transporter protein 8 (ZnT8) [1]. Classically, the initial autoantibodies that start appearing in patients with T1DM (from the age of 9–24 months) are IAA and then GADA by the age of 36 months. Most T1DM patients show multiple autoantibodies and only about 10% of patients display a single autoantibody. It was reported that the appearance of ZnT8 and IA-2A resulted in more rapid progress towards the T1DM pathology [2]. However, the most studied biomarkers, perhaps to date, are glycated haemoglobin, glycated albumin and 1,5-anhydroglucitol (1,5-AG). Judicious use of biomarkers can be quite helpful in the drug development process too. More efficient discovery and use of biomarkers in the development of anti-diabetic drugs will depend on advancing our understanding of the pathogenesis of diabetes, especially its micro- and macrovascular complications.

This chapter describes the various biomarkers for type 1 diabetes mellitus and type 2 diabetes mellitus.

BIOMARKERS FOR T1DM

As mentioned in the previous chapters, T1DM is a chronic autoimmune disease with both genetic and environmental aetiology that leads to the destruction of the functional β-cells. T1DM is primarily divided into the following stages [3]:

a) Appearance of β-cells autoantibodies (stage 1)
b) Appearance of hyperglycaemia with hypoglycaemic episodes too (stage 2)
c) Final T1DM pathology and related comorbidities (stage 3)

Before moving on to the serum biomarkers for T1DM, we must mention briefly the genetic markers. Mutation and variation in HLA genotypes are widely associated with the risk of progression of T1DM. This high risk is attributed due to the fact that the HLA genes are highly responsible for T-cell selection, antigen presentation and T-cell activation. Among the HLA alleles, *HLA DR* and *HLA DQ* class II loci are most responsible for the T1DM risk. Among these, specifically, *HLA DRB1*03, HLA DRB1*04* and *HLA DQB1*0302 (HLA DR3/4 DQ8)* impart the highest risk in the development and progression of T1DM. Apart from the HLA genotypes, two other genes, *INS* (the pro-insulin gene) and *PTPN22* (protein tyrosine phosphatase N22), also significantly increase the risk of development of T1DM. A VNTR variant of INS, INS VNTR I, is shown to be responsible for increased T1DM risk while an increase in phosphatase activity of PTP is seen in T1DM patients [4].

The most common and currently important clinical serum biomarkers for T1DM are IAA, GADA, IA-2A and ZnT8. The autoantibody theory gained importance as T1DM biomarker with the detection of ICA that is now a collective term for different T1DM associated autoantibodies. ICAs are determined in a special unit known as the Juvenile Diabetes Foundation (JDF) unit. The lowest positive value of ICA is considered to be 10 JDF. ICAs are detected in almost 80% of new-onset T1DM patients, but usually decline in due course of the disease. Approximately 5% of T1DM patients remain serologically positive for ICA in their lifetime [5, 6]. Being non-specific, ICAs are currently not recommended for diagnostic purposes [7].

Glutamic acid decarboxylase (GAD) is the enzyme responsible for the synthesis of neurotransmitter gamma amino butyric acid or GABA from glutamic acid. GABA is the primary inhibitory neurotransmitter in humans. GAD is expressed as 65 kDa (GAD65) and 67 kDa (GAD67) isoform but GAD65 acts as the autoantigen in T1DM pathology. GAD autoantibody (GADA) was first reported in patients with a rare genetic disorder known as stiff person syndrome. Later, these GADA were reported to be a primary marker in T1DM patients detected from the very onset. Unlike ICA, the serum level of GADA is found persistently in T1DM patients; therefore, it is currently more preferred than ICA for T1DM diagnosis [5]. Certain unusual findings suggest that GADA is less frequent in males below 10 years of age if they present T1DM, but the diagnostic sensitivity is approximately 80% in the older subjects of both genders. In certain striking reports, it is also observed that children born to T1DM mothers, who are GADA positive, were likely to be much less GADA positive in future, i.e. these children were found to be seronegative to GADA. This might be because due to *in utero* exposure to GADA, these children have developed immunological tolerance to the autoantibody [8]. GADA is found to be more consistent as compared to other autoantibodies in T1DM for long-term diagnosis. Because of detection of GADA in the early pre-clinical stage of T1DM and ease of detection, it is currently one of the most utilised biomarkers for T1DM diagnosis. GADA detection is also of key importance for latent autoimmune diabetes of adults or LADA (type 1.5 diabetes) since LADA patients clinically display T2DM characteristics but show seropositivity for GADA [9]. The assessment of GADA titre helps in further classification of LADA since a high titre is generally found in LADA patients with phenotypic characteristics similar to T1DM patients (LADA type 1), while a low titre is usually seen in patients with phenotypic characteristics similar to those observed in T2DM patients (LADA type 2) [10]. In an interesting finding, it was also reported that T1DM and LADA patients with high titre of GADA have a very high chance of developing autoimmune thyroid disorder. The prevalence of thyroid-specific antibodies (thyroglobulin antibody and thyroid peroxidase antibody) was almost 27% in T1DM patients and almost 21% in LADA patients with high titre of GADA. Therefore, T1DM and LADA patients with high GADA titre must have a regular thyroid function diagnosis [11]. In a recent interesting study regarding the association of structure of GAD65 and insulin dependence in diabetes patients, it was shown that the subjects having full-length GAD65 antigen were less likely to go on insulin therapy, while those with a N-terminal truncated GAD65 were more prone to go on insulin therapy. Also, a small subgroup of patients with full-length GAD65 displayed clinical phenotype similar to GADA-negative T2DM patients. Thus, the detection of autoantibodies corresponding to the full-length and truncated GAD65 is essential in predicting the progression to insulin therapy and severity of the disease [12].

Insulinoma-associated antigen-2 (IA-2) is a type 1 transmembrane protein that contains an N-terminal glycosylated extracellular region, a region spanning the plasma membrane and a C-terminal cytoplasmic portion. The antigenic epitopes of IA-2 are found entirely in the cytoplasmic region. The protein tyrosine phosphatase (PTP) like domain is the major antigenic epitope of this protein. It was reported that inhibition of IA-2 led to diminished insulin secretion and resultant elevated glucose level. IA-2 is said to work in mobilisation of insulin containing vesicles and their exocytosis [13]. IA-2As were initially found when scientists were screening certain proteins produced by insulinoma cells for their reactivity with the serum of T1DM subjects. The initial IA-2 autoantibodies were found against the intracellular domain of the protein and were known as 'ICA512' autoantibodies. Thus, the autoantibodies are referred to as IA-2A when full-length antigen is in assay, while the description of ICA512 is used when only intracellular domain is used for immunoprecipitation immunoassays [14]. IA-2A is the autoantibody against a protein-tyrosine phosphatase antigen (or insulinoma antigen-2) that is present with the insulin secretory granules in the β-cells. Because of its presence in the insulin secretory granules, IA-2 has been reported to aid in biogenesis of insulin secretory granules, insulin secretion and beta-cell expansion [15]. Along with GADA, it is an almost equally important biomarker for the diagnosis of T1DM. It was also shown to be positive in patients who displayed negative for GADA. IA-2A was reported to be more prevalent in patients with mutation in HLA-DR4 alleles. The prevalence of IA-2A was similar in subjects in both genders and all ages suffering from T1DM. As stated earlier, GADA is shown to be positive in people with autoimmune thyroid disease (or T1DM may predispose people towards such a disease) and stiff person syndrome; IA-2A is shown to be specific to T1DM patients [16]. As a direct marker for β-cells' destruction, it was also shown that children who tested positive for IA-2A at diagnosis had diminished C-peptide levels as compared to children who were IA-2A negative [17]. In another interesting, yet controversial, study, it was found that autoantibodies such as IA-2A or IAA were found to be positive mostly in patients who were GADA positive, while GADA-negative patients hardly show positivity for more than one other autoantibody [18].

Zinc transporter 8 (ZnT8) is a protein (encoded by the SLC30A8 gene from the solute link carrier 30 gene family) with six transmembrane domains and with a histidine-rich loop between the fourth and fifth domains that represents a classical feature of all ZnT proteins. Zinc transporters are a family of transmembrane proteins that are involved in the maintenance and regulation of total cellular zinc content. ZnT8 homodimers are inserted in the membrane of the insulin secretory granules, with N- and C- terminal domains facing towards the cytoplasm while the histidine-rich loop is present towards the lumen of the granules. ZnT8 play a critical role in the transport and accumulation of zinc in the secretory granules that stabilise stored insulin as tightly packed hexamers. The expression of ZnT8 in β-cells is said to increase the overall zinc content which also protects β-cells from apoptosis due to zinc depletion. ZnT8 is also said to protect the insulin-secreting β-cells from cytokine-mediated destruction. ZnT8 expression is primarily restricted to pancreatic β-cells, while very little expression is also mentioned in retinal pigment epithelium. ZnT8 autoantibody epitopes are present in the N-terminal or the C-terminal cytoplasmic domains. It was reported that less than 10% of ZnT8-positive patients have autoantibodies to the N-terminal domain, while the C-terminal domain was responsible for major proportion of the autoantibody pool. Moreover, ZnT8 autoantibodies have been identified that are specific either to the arginine or tryptophan polymorphic variants at amino acid residue 325 in the C-terminal domain [15, 19]. Because of this high specialised expression, β-cells have the highest concentration of zinc among all the cells of the human body. And in β-cells, almost 70% of the zinc ions are located in the insulin-secretory vesicles. Apart from its role in stabilising the hexameric conformation of insulin inside the secretory granules, zinc has also been reported to have an important role in the processing of proinsulin. Another important fact related to zinc and diabetes is that zinc ions prevent the formation of islet amyloid polypeptide (IAPP). IAPP precursor is co-formed and co-secreted from the insulin secretory granules, and formation of IAPP (a misfolded protein) is found to have a great effect on the development of diabetes [20]. In a recent study conducted in India, it was reported that the prevalence of ZnT8 as a T1DM marker was more pronounced than IA-2A and the combined diagnosis of GADA and ZnT8 displayed more accuracy in detecting T1DM. In newly diagnosed T1DM cases, the prevalence of ZnT8 was almost 45% [21]. In a detailed review on major autoantibodies related to T1DM, it was stated that in young patients with new-onset T1DM, 63% were found to be positive for the ZnT8 autoantibody (vs. 72% positive for GADA, 68% positive for IA-2A and 55% positive for IAA). Even in young patients with new-onset T1DM who were found to be negative for GADA, IA-2A or IAA, 26% resulted positive for the ZnT8 autoantibody. The addition of the ZnT8 autoantibody to the pool of T1DM biomarkers led to more precise diagnosis of the disease and increased the percentage of diagnosed patients (5.8% found negative in new-onset T1DM with GADA, IAA and IA-2A vs. 1.8% found negative when ZnT8 autoantibody was added) [5]. In view of pancreatic transplantation, it was recently reported that the addition of ZnT8 autoantibodies along with GADA and IA-2A increased the detection of transplantation failure. Thus, the introduction of the ZnT8 autoantibody to the marker profile increased the sensitivity and specificity of diagnosis of post-transplantation failure in patients requiring a pancreas/islet transplant [22].

Insulin autoantibodies (IAA), as the name suggests, are the autoantibodies against one of the major hormones responsible for glucose regulation. The epitopes on the IAAs have been indirectly characterised using various recombinant insulin or insulin analogues. IAAs generally do not interact or bind to the denatured insulin. The primary amino acid residues required for binding of high affinity IAAs are found to be located within residues 8–13 in the A chain of insulin, while most of the low affinity IAAs are shown to interact within residues 28–30 of the B chain of the insulin. Specific experimental investigations have reported that IAAs that interact with A chain residues numbered 8–13 can bind pro-insulin too, but such a trend is not seen with B chain residues numbered 28–30 [15]. The IAAs are relevant only at the diagnosis of new-onset of diabetes in younger children. Once the exogenous therapeutic insulin is administered, it can anyway elicit the antibody generation and the exact quantification of IAAs is diluted [5].

BIOMARKERS FOR T2DM

Since blood glucose (fasting glucose and post-prandial glucose) measurement is the most common determinant for T2DM, this section will deal with biomarkers that are indicative of the progress of T2DM. Such common biomarkers are glycated haemoglobin (HbA1c), glycated albumin (GlyAlb) and 1,5-anhydroglucitol (1,5-AG). This section will also deal with uric acid as a 'possible' biomarker for diabetes and its metabolism.

Glycated Haemoglobin (HbA1c)

As per the available scientific records, the first description of glycated haemoglobin (HbA1c) is found in a work by Rahbar at University of Tehran, Iran. He found an electrophoretically fast moving abnormal haemoglobin variant in two patients who were suffering from type 2 diabetes mellitus [23]. As discussed in a previous chapter, glycated haemoglobin is a haemoglobin variant that is produced as a result on glycation (non-enzymatic addition of glucose moieties) of haemoglobin. A high value of HbA1c shows that the person is suffering from diabetes. Although HbA1c is also used to keep a tap on the glucose fluctuations and progress of T1DM, this section will mainly deal with T2DM, and 'diabetes' henceforth in this section will mean T2DM. HbA1c is currently treated as the 'gold standard' marker for diagnosing diabetes, while also checking the progression and condition of the disease. Initial structural examination of glycated haemoglobin, in particular the HbA1c fraction as analysed on cation exchange chromatography, qualitatively demonstrated that the glycation occurred at the N-terminus of the β-chain of the haemoglobin. Glycaemic control or fluctuations over the last 3 to 4 months can be examined by determining the ratio of glycated to non-glycated haemoglobin [24]. Though ADA also recommends the use of HbA1c along with fasting glucose and OGTT, there seems to be certain basic problems with the use of HbA1c. HbA1c represents only a fraction of haemoglobin that has become glycated. Secondly, this fraction represents only the protein which is exclusively found in RBCs and nowhere else in the body. Thirdly, the movement of glucose in and out of RBCs can also vary from person to person along with the RBC turnover. Also, a number of blood disorders and haemoglobinopathies might not give the true expected value. For example, a common condition of anaemia due to iron deficiency can, for reasons unexplained, result in an increase in HbA1c by 1–1.5% that subsequently reduces following iron supplementation. Therefore, depending solely on HbA1c for diagnosis and therapeutic purposes does not seem to be logical. But, contrary to this logic and report, an analysis of the National Health and Nutrition Examination Survey (NHANES), USA data showed that 50–60% of patients with fasting plasma glucose (FPG) ≥7 mmol/L had HbA1c ≤6.5%, suggesting that HbA1c might be beneficial in decreasing the number of people wrongly diagnosed as having diabetes [25]. But this could probably be explained by the fact that fasting plasma glucose gives the most recent value of glucose control (after overnight fasting of 8–10 hours), while HbA1c is considered an average value. Thus, a person might have increased FPG (probably due to diet or stress or medication) but might show a normal HbA1c value. Secondly, the status of haemoglobin depends upon a variety of factors such as the number of RBCs, ethnicity, geographical location and dietary patterns. Thus, using HbA1c as the gold standard does not seems logical and accurate in predicting diabetes, though it has been reported that increased value of HbA1c provides a positive correlation to the cardiovascular diseases related to diabetes. Just to repeat the diagnostic criteria (mentioned in previous chapters too), a value greater than 6.5% ($\geq$48 mmol/mol) is an indication of diabetes, while the values between 5.7% to 6.4% (39–46 mmol/mol) predict the pre-diabetes stage. Since HbA1c, FPG, IFG, and OGTT have their individual importance in the diagnosis of diabetes, no single criterion could be determined as 'best' for diagnosing diabetes. The criteria values should always be correlated with the clinical characteristics [26]. In terms of patient compliance, HbA1c is best suited as patients need not fast before giving the sample and the sample can be provided at any time of the day. Seeing the relation between HbA1c and cardiovascular disease prediction, it was reported that the increase in the HbA1c value indicated pronounced future cardiovascular diseases (CVDs). Thus, addition of HbA1c in regular diabetes tests could help predict the course and graph of CVDs [27]. Even for diabetes-related kidney complications and retinopathy, it was shown that there was a direct correlation between the HbA1c value and the incident microvascular pathological progression to nephropathy and retinopathy, even in the absence of clinical diabetes. Though in the case of retinopathy, hypertension was a major culprit even before a clinical rise in blood glucose [28].

Regarding the basic biology of HbA1c, normal human adult haemoglobin has three major variants, namely HbA (almost 97%), HbA2 (almost 2.5%) and HbF (0.5%). The non-enzymatic addition of glucose moieties, known as the Maillard reaction, occurs in many proteins including haemoglobin. Following the experiment by Rahbar, as mentioned earlier, researchers revealed that a hexose molecule is attached to the valine residue present at the N-terminal of the β-chain of HbA and this fraction was termed HbA1c. Years later, the International Union of Pure and Applied Chemistry (IUPAC) defined HbA1c as the fraction of the β-chain of haemoglobin that has a stable hexose moiety on the valine residue at the N-terminal. Apart from the mentioned location above, glycation in haemoglobin can occur at other sites too, such as valine residue at the N-terminal of α-chain and lysine residues of both the chains. But these variants are termed glycated HbA_0. The potential value of HbA1c in diabetes diagnosis was mentioned by the WHO back in 1985, while the ADA first made its recommendation in routine semi-annual diagnosis in 1988. For measurement of HbA1c, various techniques have been used that include those based on charge differences (ion-exchange chromatography, high-performance liquid chromatography or HPLC, electrophoresis and isoelectric focusing), structural differences basis (affinity chromatography and immunoassay) and photochemical analysis (spectrophotometry). While other methods have become obsolete, the most widely used methods today are those based on HPLC and immunoassay. Currently, there are more than 100 reported measurement protocols for the quantification of HbA1c, Thus, their standardisation was necessary to get similar reporting. To get a hold on this, the American Association of Clinical Chemistry (AACC) created a committee known as the National Glycohemoglobin Standardization Program or NGSP in 1993 that is currently the standardisation authority for testing HbA1c. Apart from NGSP, another standardisation committee was formed by the International Federation of Clinical Chemistry and Laboratory Medicine (IFCC) which recommended a separate method of estimating HbA1c. But due to its time consuming, technically demanding and expensive nature, the protocol is not widely accepted in terms of laboratory and patient compliance for routine sample analysis. It has, though, been set as a reference protocol. And according to common consensus, the units and values for both NGSP and IFCC have been validated and approved to be used interchangeably. In 2004, the American Diabetes Association (ADA), the European Association for the Study of

Table 5.1 Comparison between NGSP and IFCC Measurement of HbA1c Values

NGSP (%)	IFCC (mmol/mol)
4.0	20
5.0	31
6.0	42
6.5	48
7.0	53
8.0	64
9.0	75
10.0	86
11.0	97
12.0	108

Glycated albumin (GA).

Diabetes (EASD) and the International Diabetes Federation (IDF) have reached a common harmonisation status for HbA1c reporting. As per this agreement, HbA1c worldwide should be reported in NGSP-IFCC units (both in % and mmol/mol units). This conversion value has been derived based on a the NGSP-IFCC 'master equation', that is [NGSP = 0.09148(IFCC) + 2.152] or [IFCC = 10.93(NGSP) − 23.50]. Table 5.1 above describes the comparative values of NGSP and IFCC for HbA1c diagnosis [29].

As seen above, there are instances and pathophysiological conditions where glycated haemoglobin measurement cannot be considered. For such cases, other diabetes markers could be considered. One widely studied marker is glycated albumin (GA). Albumin is a 66.7 kDa large protein composed of a single polypeptide chain with 585 amino acid residues. In humans, albumin is the primary plasma protein with an almost 60% share of all plasma proteins, with a normal value between 3 g/dL and 5 g/dL. It is produced by the liver and plays a crucial role in maintaining oncotic pressure, pH of plasma, binding and transport of drugs, metals and various hormones. Though there are 59 lysine residues in albumin that are prone to glycation much more so than other residues, the lysine at position 525 is most prone to glycation. The whole pool of glycated plasma proteins is collectively known as 'fructosamine' and by virtue of its abundance, glycated albumin (GA) is considered to be the most abundant fructosamine that represents almost 80% of total glycation in the human plasma. Since plasma proteins, as compared to intracellular proteins, are more exposed to the blood glucose, they have a better and stronger chance of being glycated. Thus, for an equal amount of glucose concentration, the rate of GA formation and amount of concentration of GA will always be higher than HbA1c. Like HbA1c, GA can also be estimated by HPLC, immunoassay, boronate affinity chromatography, colorimetric assay using thiobarbituric acid and enzymatic method using ketamine oxidase, though most of these methods are seldom used clinically. Even when not used in routine clinical evaluation for diabetes, GA can be treated as a better alternative to HbA1c in cases where there is a confirmed change in the patient's haemoglobin. It was reported that conditions such as haemolytic anaemia and bleeding episodes result in decreased HbA1c values, while iron deficiency anaemia, thalassaemia and haemoglobinopathies resulted in its increment. In regard to gestational diabetes, it was reported that there were significant changes in HbA1c estimation due to various physiological demands in different gestational stages, while GA was found to be stable throughout the gestational period. In diabetic patients who develop chronic kidney disease (CKD), HbA1c may not be considered a reliable biomarker since the CKD state presents a lot of complications that alter the RBC and haemoglobin state. Patients with CKD usually suffer from erythropoietin deficiency that leads to the development of anaemia. Since erythropoietin is synthesised by the kidney, therefore, it is very often necessary to use exogenous therapeutic erythropoietin to compensate the reduced endogenous synthesis. The iron level is also often seen to be altered in the case of diabetic CKD which results in iron deficiency anaemia, too. Further, because of persistent and deteriorating anaemic state, these patients may require frequent blood transfusion. Also, haemodialysis often results in 20–50% diminished lifespan of the RBCs that also contribute to the false values of HbA1c. But since the case of CKD also presents increased proteinuria, GA assay could also result in false analysis. Thus, careful analysis must be carried out to choose the better marker among the two in the case of CKD patients. Moreover, as the half-life of albumin is shorter than RBCs (20 *vs.* 120), GA estimation could be a better diabetes marker for short-term goals and diagnoses. Since albumin remains in direct contact with the plasma glucose, logically the effect of anti-diabetic therapy could be better evaluated by estimating GA rather than HbA1c. Though with all the stated benefits, GA analysis could still be misleading in certain pathological conditions such as hyperthyroidism, hypothyroidism and hepatic disorders such as cirrhosis. Theoretically, any condition that can alter the production, distribution or metabolism of albumin could falsely implicate GA values [30, 31]. In terms of evaluation of CVDs, GA has been reported to be a more reliable marker than HbA1c as it correlated better with the incidences and severity of CVDs with better glycaemic fluctuations. Also due to a shorter half-life compared to HbA1c, GA could be more sensitive and lead to early diagnosis. Moreover, GA has been reported to be directly involved in the atherosclerotic process. Therefore, its estimation could guide us better for CVDs [32]. The Japanese Society for Dialysis Therapy (JSDT) presents the best practice guide for diabetic patients on haemodialysis and suggested GA <20.0% as the clinical target for glycaemic control in such patients without a known history of CVDs, while the value was set at <24.0% for those with CVDs. In a very recent study to figure out a relationship between GA value and 1-year mortality rate in diabetic patients undergoing haemodialysis, it was reported that the 1-year mortality in such patients was least corresponding to a GA value between 15.6% and 18.2% and the trend was linear in nature [33]. GA has been reported to be a better indicator of glycaemic fluctuations than HbA1c in diabetic patients with improper diabetes control. As uncontrolled post-prandial hyperglycaemia is more responsible than fasting hyperglycaemia for CVDs, GA is considered better biomarker compared to HbA1c for diabetes-associated CVD. In an aged population with diminished muscle biochemistry, the post-prandial muscle glucose regulation is hampered. As a result of this uncontrolled mechanism, the aged diabetic population experiences post-prandial hyperglycaemia at a much higher rate than the younger subjects. Therefore, GA is said to be a better glycaemic marker as compared to HbA1c in such a population [34].

1,5-Anhydroglucitol (1,5-AG)

When talking of alternate biomarkers in the diagnosis of diabetes, 1,5-anhydroglucitol (1,5-AG) has recently attracted worldwide interest in being simple and directly related to a particular glycaemic threshold, primarily post-prandial fluctuations. 1,5-AG is a dietary monosaccharide that is chemically 1-deoxyglucose. The comparative structure of glucose and 1,5-AG is given below in Figure 5.1.

1,5-AG was first reported in plants around 1888, while its presence in humans was first reported in 1972. It is absorbed in the body through our plant-based diets. It is found to be particularly high in soybeans. Because of the structural similarity with glucose, its renal proximal tubular reabsorption is competitively inhibited by glucose molecules. Most of the 1,5-AG (99.9%) gets reabsorbed from renal tubules in normal physiological state, while in diabetic state, its concentration in urine increases (due to glucose mediated competitive inhibition) that results in a decrease in plasma 1,5-AG levels. 1,5-AG serum levels among a healthy population show a wide range (12–40 mg/ml), where males show a significantly higher value than their female counterparts. Because 1,5-AG is metabolically inert and is highly reabsorbed from the renal tubules, its plasma level is mostly consistent throughout the day in healthy individuals. The renal glucose threshold is that concentration of serum glucose above which the glucose starts appearing in the urine because the kidney has a limit of glucose reabsorption. This value has been calculated between 160 mg/dL and 190 mg/dL. Thus, in simple words, when there is a persistent hyperglycaemia, the high glucose leads to inhibition of renal 1,5-AG reabsorption and, thus, both glucose and 1,5-AG appears in urine. In this case of hyperglycaemia, while the plasma glucose is high, the plasma 1,5-AG decreases significantly. Whereas HbA1c (average of a 120-day period) and fructosamine (2-week period) takes time to develop and show an extended glucose fluctuation, the direct reabsorption antagonism between glucose and 1,5-AG in the renal proximal tubule throughout the day and the instant decrease of the plasma 1,5-AG level following raised plasma glucose levels provide a knowledge of average glycaemia over a prolonged time period in a single measurement, while repeated measurements demonstrate fluctuation in plasma glucose levels over a much shorter time period. Encashing the diagnostic value of 1,5-AG, Japan has developed the world's first commercial kit for measurement of 1,5-AG that is available under the name Glycomark™. It was initially approved in Japan and the United States and trials in various countries are ongoing [35]. The variation in 1,5-AG depends on the period and extent of glycosuria, and 1,5-AG is found to recover at a rate of approximately

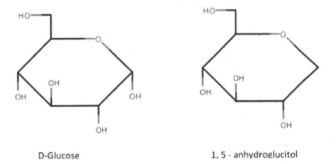

D-Glucose   1, 5 - anhydroglucitol

Figure 5.1 A comparative figure of glucose and 1,5-AG.

0.3 µg/ml/day when the normoglycaemic condition is restored. Therefore, 1,5-AG is very sensitive towards glycaemic condition reflecting an even transitory boost in glucose within a few days. Attributed to this sensitivity, 1,5-AG is considered a better marker for post-prandial glucose fluctuations. It was speculated in a major patient-centric study more than a decade ago that in clinical practice, HbA1c and 1,5-AG could be accessed sequentially; first, HbA1c assay could be performed to identify diabetic patients who have moderately or well controlled glycaemic condition (HbA1c value 6.5–8.0%) and then the 1,5-AG assay could follow to determine the magnitude of post-prandial glucose fluctuations. If the HbA1c value is found to be elevated but the 1,5-AG is normal, basal glycaemia targeting treatments may prove to be more useful. On the other hand, if HbA1c is increased and 1,5-AG is decreased, a post-prandial hyperglycaemia-targeted treatment approach could be more fruitful [36]. Another interesting study reported in 2010 reveals that 1,5-AG can differentiate between two major sub-types of MODY (HNF1A and GK) and with other types of diabetes (T1DM and T2DM). Biochemical markers that can aptly differentiate among such diabetes types could prove to be very useful clinically. The HNF1A mutation type MODY shows a reduced renal glucose threshold due to decreased expression of SGLT-2. It was found that the 1,5-AG level was highest in the GK-mutation MODY patients, while it was significantly low and quite similar in HNF1A type, T1DM and T2DM. Though the levels were very close in HNF1A and T1DM patients [37]. A recent study has also revealed a strong association of 1,5-AG with diabetes-mediated microvascular complications. Lower values of 1,5-AG strongly indicated development of diabetic retinopathy and chronic kidney disease [38]. In another study aiming to associate 1,5-AG with atherosclerotic characteristics in diabetic patients, researchers found a strong negative association of 1,5-AG with plaque score, as determined by ultrasonography imaging, even when the HbA1c was below the threshold of 6.5% [39]. Similar recent patient-based studies supported the fact that since post-prandial glucose excursion is a high-risk factor for development of CVDs, 1,5-AG could serve as a better marker to predict the CVD and related outcome as compared to the traditional HbA1c. They also pointed out the essential fact that since the level of 1,5-AG remains constant throughout the day, a fasting sample is not required which becomes a better criterion as per the patient compliance. Moreover, the importance of 1,5-AG diagnosis is also evident from the fact that it was shown to be significantly associated with the development of major cardiovascular complications even in the non-diabetic population without any previous CVDs. Thus, this marker is evident to be a strong predictor of CVDs in non-diabetic patients with no previous history of CVDs [40, 41]. In patients with percutaneous coronary interventions (PCI; commonly known as coronary stenting), lower 1,5-AG was significantly associated with future development of clinical cardiovascular complications [42]. A very recent study also supported the fact and revealed that 1,5-AG was significantly lower in patients who died of acute coronary syndrome and this could be used to predict the long-term mortality in patients showing clinical symptoms for acute coronary syndrome even when the HbA1c is less than 7% [43].

Uric Acid

Uric acid is a by-product of purine metabolism that is produced in the liver and primarily excreted by the renal system and intestines. Uric acid is an excellent antioxidant and perhaps responsible for almost 75% of plasma anti-oxidant activity; however, an increase in levels of serum uric acid (SUA) increases the chances of developing metabolic syndrome characterised by hypertriglyceridaemia, insulin resistance, high inflammatory markers and increase risk of cardiovascular events. Although it is said that a chronic elevated SUA is harmful, an acute increase in SUA could be a protective mechanism [44]. A study by Dehghan et al. published in 2008 shows that increased SUA is an independent risk factor for development of diabetes and that chronically high SUA also resulted in increased oxidative stress and high inflammatory TNF-α, while a recent study by Wang et al. also confirmed the similar result that higher SUA is associated with higher fasting plasma glucose and risk for development of future metabolic syndrome [45, 46]. Several studies, though, published contradictory results that SUA has an inverse relationship to the blood sugar level and HbA1c [47]. Hyperuricaemia (increased uric acid in the blood) has been suggested as a novel risk factor for diabetes. The levels of uric acid in an individual is a combined result of genetic factors and a multitude of lifestyle-related factors such as food habits, exercise, work type and means of transportation. Uric acid's definite role in this prevalent disease is still the subject of much discussion because it is always accompanied with other major risk factors such as obesity and high visceral adiposity; hence, there have been projects to relate them all.

Coming back to uric acid levels, the introduction of diets rich in sugar and purines led to a remarkable rise in serum uric acid and a widespread increase in obesity and diabetes. Elevated serum uric acid consistently predicts the development of obesity and diabetes. Lowering serum uric acid prevents insulin resistance in fructose-dependent and fructose-independent animal models of metabolic syndrome. A pilot randomised clinical study reported that lowering uric acid with a uricosuric agent improves insulin resistance, and a randomised trial showed that lowering uric acid with allopurinol also improves insulin resistance in hyperuricaemic individuals. Cellular mechanisms by which uric acid can induce diabetes have been identified. However, currently, controlled clinical trials to determine whether lowering serum uric acid can slow the development of metabolic syndrome and diabetes are in progress. Uric acid is the end product of purine metabolism. Uric acid can act as a pro-oxidant, particularly at increased concentration, and may, therefore, be a marker of oxidative stress. Increased levels of uric acid have been associated with insulin resistance and established T2DM [48]. Dehghan et al. have demonstrated that uric acid is an independent predictor of incident T2DM in the general population [45]. Uric acid cannot simply be viewed as a secondary phenomenon. Uric acid and its changes during follow-up were related to corresponding changes in fasting and post-load glucose and insulin levels [48]. The present project is a population-based demographic study that tries to, firstly, compare the serum uric acid levels in the type 2 diabetics and controls, and, secondly, to correlate various diabetic parameters with the serum uric acid levels in the patients and controls. The public health impact of high serum uric acid may be greater than what is currently thought. Uric acid is neither a target for treatment in asymptomatic hyperuricaemia nor a risk marker in clinical practice and even the methods for assessment of serum uric acid are widely available and inexpensive. Hence measurement of serum uric acid levels could play a valuable role as a predictor marker in early type 2 diabetics as well as a potent antioxidant therapeutic [48].

Uric acid is able to react with different free radicals forming a relatively stable urate radical and thus stopping radical reactions. Uric acid can act as a pro-oxidant and it may thus be a marker of oxidative stress indicating pre-diabetes, but it may also have a therapeutic role as an antioxidant. Urate, the soluble form of uric acid, can scavenge the superoxide and the hydroxyl radicals and it can chelate the transition metals [49]. Hyperuricaemia has also been added to the set of metabolic abnormalities which are associated with insulin resistance and/or hyperinsulinaemia in metabolic syndrome [50].

While an increase in the uric acid levels in pre-diabetes and diabetes was demonstrated by some studies, a declining trend of the serum uric acid levels with increasing blood glucose levels was observed by other research workers. The plasma urate level in humans is considerably higher than the ascorbate level, making it one of the major antioxidants in humans. Uric acid is special in the sense that it is the best antioxidant within the physiological range, but it acts as an effective pro-oxidant when there is hyperuricaemia. This is the reason why hyperuricaemia is positively associated with CVDs and metabolic syndrome. The cells, upon encountering increased uric acid, start generating reactive oxygen species (ROS) and reactive nitrogen species (RNS). This is accompanied by impaired nitric oxide generation [50].

Uric acid, a weak organic acid with a pKa of 5.75, is present principally as monosodium urate (MSU) at physiological pH values. Whereas in humans and the great apes uric acid is the end product of purine degradation, in other mammals, it is further degraded into allantoin by uricase, an enzyme that is mutated in humans and primates. The gene encoding uricase underwent mutational silencing during hominid evolution. The consequence of uricase inactivation is the appearance of urate levels that are much higher in humans ($\approx$240–360 µM) in comparison to other mammals ($\approx$30–50 µM in mice). It has been proposed that higher serum levels of urate may be of selective advantage in the evolution of hominids because of their anti-oxidant effects [51]. On the other hand, hyperuricaemia is associated with multiple diseases in humans and points to the deleterious effects of high concentrations of urate [52]. Figure 5.2 shows a basic uric acid biosynthesis pathway.

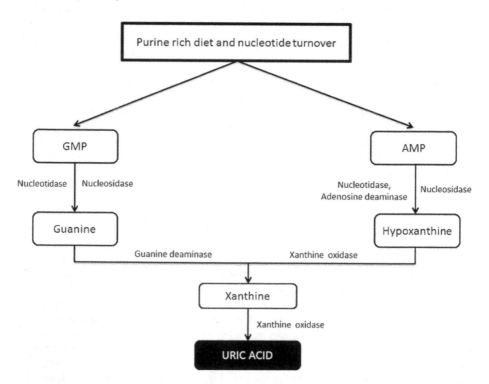

Figure 5.2 Pathways of uric acid biosynthesis.

Serum uric acid (SUA) has been predicted to be an independent factor for T2DM in many studies. Alloxan has long been used in experimental models to induce diabetes by destroying β-cells and it was shown that alloxan-like metabolites derived from uric acid oxidation could lead to similar consequences in humans too, resulting in decreased glucose-stimulated insulin secretion [52]. Another meta-analysis reported a positive correlation between SUA and impaired fasting glucose (IFG) and T2DM [53]. Uric acid has been reported to worsen the insulin resistance in animal models by inhibiting nitric oxide (NO) which is essential for glucose mediated insulin release and insulin mediated glucose uptake [53, 54]. It was reported in a meta-analysis that each 1 mg/dL increment in SUA resulted in a 17% increased chance of T2DM along with an increase in parameters of metabolic syndrome like triglyceride and hypertension [53]. A finding also stated that hyperuricaemia results in increased oxidative stress and TNF-α production, which in turn increase the insulin resistance [54]. Another Indian study found that SUA linearly increased with an increase in serum insulin level and glycated haemoglobin level (HbA1c), indicating a high incidence of insulin resistance with an increment in SUA [55]. In early animal studies, it was found that high uric acid might result in the inhibition of glucose-stimulated insulin secretion (GSIS) by binding to an arginine residue on the β-cells [56].

During the production of uric acid catalysed by xanthine-oxidase (XO), ROS are generated as a by-product, which have a significant role in the increased vascular oxidative stress. XO is a hepatic enzyme which catalyses the production of uric acid, nitric oxide and reactive oxygen species, which potentially damage deoxyribonucleic acid, ribonucleic acid and proteins, inactivate enzymes, oxidise amino acids and convert poly-unsaturated fatty acids to lipids. Reduction of molecular oxygen by either form of the enzyme yields superoxide and hydrogen peroxide. UA is the most abundant aqueous antioxidant in humans, and contributes as much as two-thirds to all free radical scavenging capacity in plasma. It is particularly effective in quenching hydroxyl, superoxide and peroxynitrite radicals, and may serve a protective physiological role by preventing lipid peroxidation. In a variety of organs and vascular beds, local UA concentrations increase during acute oxidative stress, and the increased concentrations might be a compensatory mechanism that confers protection against increased free radical activity [57, 58]. The relative hyperuricaemia in humans has raised questions about its evolutionary advantages, and its association with diseases requires understanding of how it can become deleterious at high concentrations as well as in lower concentrations. The anti-oxidant activity of uric acid can prevent peroxynitrite-induced protein nitrosation, lipid and protein peroxidation, and inactivation of tetrahydrobiopterin, a cofactor necessary for NOS. Uric acid also protects LDL (low density lipoprotein) from Cu^{2+} mediated oxidation [58]. In a recent meta-analysis, it was observed that there is a positive correlation between SUA, impaired fasting glucose and T2DM [59]. On the level of diet-induced hyperuricaemia, it is an established fact that high fructose consumption results in a chronic and significant rise in serum uric acid that further leads to the complications of metabolic syndrome.

Chromogranin A

Though the consensus is that chromogranin A is a diabetes marker, we would like to briefly present this possibly interesting marker in the case of diabetes. Chromogranin A (CgA) is an acidic glycoprotein originally found in the chromaffin cells of adrenal medulla. It belongs to a family of secretory proteins collectively known as 'granins' that are present in both normal and tumour cells of neuroendocrine tissues. Usually, CgA is co-secreted with the hormone that is released from the parent cell. It has been revealed that the intracellular and/or extracellular proteolysis of CgA results in peptide fragments of various lengths that have an effect upon the cardiovascular system, angiogenesis, immunity and metabolism. It was first described by O'Connor and Bernstein that CgA could be used as a strong biomarker for various neuroendocrine tumours. But with progressing research, it was found that CgA was found to be elevated in patients with certain cardiovascular ailments, gastrointestinal disorders and certain inflammatory diseases. Human CgA is a 48 kDa 439-residue-long protein that expresses in gastrointestinal tracts (GIT), the pancreas, thyroid, adenohypophysis, neurohypophysis, atrial and ventricular cardiomyocytes and lymphoid organs. Thus, CgA-derived polypeptide fragments have been shown to have important biological effects on these physiological systems. These polypeptide fragments are large fragments lacking the C-terminal region, and shorter polypeptide fragments such as CgA_{1-76} (vasostatin-I), CgA_{1-113} (vasostatin-II), CgA_{79-113} (vasoconstrictive-inhibitory factor, VIF), $CgA_{250-301}$ (pancreastatin), $CgA_{352-372}$ (catestatin) and $CgA_{411-436}$ (serpinin), mentioned in order of numerical fragmentation. Among these fragments, for example, pancreastatin or $CgA_{250-301}$ (as per the scope of this book) is shown to inhibit insulin secretion and has an important regulatory role in glucose and lipid metabolism. Though there is a debate on the normal plasma level of CgA in normal humans, it has been reported to be somewhere between 0.5–5 nM [60].

In *in vitro* and animal experiments, it was found that pancreastatin inhibited the glucose-induced insulin secretion (GSIS) by suppressing the increase in Ca^{2+} in β-cells. Moreover, it stimulated the release of glucagon in such animals that resulted in the inhibition of insulin-stimulated glycogenesis in the liver and promoted glycogenolysis. In adipocytes too, pancreastatin inhibited the insulin-stimulated glucose uptake and metabolism while inducing lipolysis. Its concentration was shown to be elevated in humans suffering from hypertension, and T2DM [61, 62]. Schmid et al. [63] demonstrated a decade ago that betagranin, an N-terminal 21 kDa fragment from CgA, is a part of insulin granules and inhibits the insulin secretion in response to glucose flux in rats and mice pancreatic cell lines and *in vivo* models – an effect similar to that of pancreastatin. But the presence and mention of betagranin in humans is debatable, as per the literature review done by the authors. The first strong evidence that CgA might be involved as an autoantigen in T1DM comes from the work of Stadinski et al. in 2010 [64]. The team demonstrated that WE14, a 14-residue fragment of CgA, functions as a strong autoantigen for CD4+ T-cells, which results in their activation leading to an autoimmune condition. This result, however, was obtained in non-obese diabetic (NOD) mice models. In 2014, Gottlieb et al. [65] reported that CgA is an autoantigen for T-cells in T1DM human patients. The team demonstrated that, similar to that in NOD mice, the WE14 fragment from CgA also serves as a strong autoantigen in new-onset T1DM in humans. In the case of T2DM, it was reported in two cross-sectional studies that the plasma CgA was significantly increased in T2DM patients than in non-diabetic controls. However, careful observation is required for CgA detection as higher levels have been seen in other pathological conditions such as various cancers, hepatic cirrhosis, hepatitis, pancreatitis, *Helicobacter pylori* infection (related gastric ulcer), inflammatory bowel syndrome (IBS) and a few more. Thus, detecting CgA in diabetic patients must have exclusion criteria with the above-mentioned diseases or should be carefully correlated [61]. Therefore, to date, CgA has been seen as a common marker for both T1DM and T2DM. But as per better empirical evidence with regards to T1DM, we can hypothesise that higher CgA in T2DM patients might render them vulnerable to gradual and further β-cell loss as the disease progresses.

Skin and Lens Autofluorescence

Skin autofluorescence (SAF) has been reported to be caused by the accumulation of AGEs, and is thus considered an important diagnostic marker in diabetes, though not widely used for diagnosis. SAF is considered a measurement of collagen-based AGE formation resulting in fluorescence. SAF has been seen to be an important marker in predicting diabetes-related renal pathology. SAF has been positively related to mortality in patients with uncontrolled diabetes. Since renal clearance of AGEs decreases with progressing renal damage, accumulation state predicts the renal condition along with other damaging effects of AGEs. Since AGEs are one of the major causative agents of diabetes complications, the non-invasive SAF measurement is highly useful in predicting the diabetes progression and therapeutic outcome. It has been reported that SAF measurement can be a useful marker for predicting and diagnosing the progression of microvascular complications, but has hardly any diagnostic value in diabetic retinopathy [66]. Secondly, in another study on diabetic patients, it was observed that SAF was positively correlated with hypertension, increased plasma triglyceride and decreased HDL that are components of metabolic syndrome [67]. Apart from SAF, ocular lens autofluorescence (LAF) has been reported to be another useful non-invasive marker for predicting the severity of diabetes. Persistent hyperglycaemia has been linked to an increased LAF. But lack of diagnostic instruments resulted in its limited use in diagnosis of diabetes. Recently, Freedom Meditech, Inc. United States, has received U.S. Food and Drug Administration (USFDA) approval to market scanning confocal bimicroscope to measure LAF without pupil dilation. Increased LAF has been shown to be positively correlated to diabetic retinopathy. LAF has recently been reported to be used even for undiagnosed T2DM [68]. Apart from lens autofluorescence in diabetes, corneal and retinal autofluorescence has also been reported to be strongly related to the progression of diabetes [69]. A recent report on 191 subjects also supported the facts that LAF can be utilised as a very useful diagnostic marker to keep a tab on the progress of diabetes [70]. The usefulness of SAF and LAF was limited mainly due to instrumental constraints. Development of more sensitive instruments can boost the use of such non-invasive diabetes markers.

REFERENCES

1. Bonifacio E. Predicting type 1 diabetes Using Biomarkers. *Diabetes Care* 2015;38(6):989–996.
2. Regnell SE, Lernmark A. Early prediction of autoimmune (type 1) diabetes. *Diabetologia* 2017;60(8):1370–1381.
3. Insel RA, Dunne JL, Atkinson MA, Chiang JL, Dabelea D, Gottlieb PA et al. Staging presymptomatic type 1 diabetes: A scientific statement of JDRF, the Endocrine Society, and the American Diabetes Association. *Diabetes Care* 2015;38(10):1964–1974.
4. Ziegler AG, Nepom GT. Prediction and pathogenesis in type 1 diabetes. *Immunity* 2010;32(4):468–478.
5. Winter WE, Schatz DA. Autoimmune markers in diabetes. *Clin Chem* 2011;57(2):168–175.
6. Taplin CE, Barker JM. Autoantibodies in type 1 diabetes. *Autoimmunity* 2008;41(1):11–18.

7. Mishra S. Pancreatic autoantibodies: Who to test and how to interpret the results. *Pract Diab* 2017;34(6):221–223.
8. Pihoker C, Gilliam LK, Hampe CS, Lernmark A. Autoantibodies in diabetes. *Diabetes* 2005;54(Suppl. 2):S52–S61.
9. Towns R, Pietropaolo M. GAD65 autoantibodies and its role as biomarker of type 1 diabetes and Latent Autoimmune Diabetes in Adults (LADA). *Drugs Future* 2011;36(11):847.
10. Liu L, Li X, Xiang Y, Huang G, Lin J, Yang L et al. Latent autoimmune diabetes in adults With low-titer GAD antibodies: Similar disease progression with type 2 diabetes. *Diabetes Care* 2015;38(1):16–21.
11. Jin P, Huang G, Lin J, Yang L, Xiang B, Zhou W et al. High titre of antiglutamic acid decarboxylase autoantibody is a strong predictor of the development of thyroid autoimmunity in patients with type 1 diabetes and latent autoimmune diabetes in adults. *Clin Endocrinol* 2011;74(5):587–592.
12. Achenbach P, Hawa MI, Krause S, Lampasona V, Jerram ST, Williams AJK et al. Autoantibodies to N-terminally truncated GAD improve clinical phenotyping of individuals with adult-onset diabetes: Action LADA 12. *Diabetologia* 2018 12;61(7):1644–1649.
13. Kim SJ, Jeong DG, Jeong SK, Yoon TS, Ryu SE. Crystal structure of the major diabetes autoantigeninsulinoma-associated protein 2 reveals distinctive immune epitopes. *Diabetes* 2007;56(1):41–48.
14. Accessed at www.mlo-online.com/the-clinical-application-of-islet-autoantibody-testing-for-the-diagnosis-of-autoimmune-diabetes.php.
15. Lampasona V, Liberati D. Islet autoantibodies. *Curr Diab Rep* 2016;16(6):53.
16. Savola K, Bonifacio E, Sabbah E, Kulmala P, Vahasalo P, Karjalainen J et al. IA-2 antibodies - A sensitive marker of IDDM with clinical onset in childhood and adolescence. *Diabetologia* 1998;41(4):424–429.
17. Sabbah E, Savola K, Kulmala P, Veijola R, Vahasalo P, Karjalainen J et al. Diabetes-associated autoantibodies in relation to clinical characteristics and natural course in children with newly diagnosed type 1 diabetes. *J Clin Endocrinol Metab* 1999;84(5):1534 –1539.
18. Kawasaki E, Nakamura K, Kuriya G, Satoh T, Kuwahara H, Kobayashi M et al. Autoantibodies to insulin, insulinoma-associated antigen-2, and zinc transporter 8 improve the prediction of early insulin requirement in adult-onset autoimmune diabetes. *J Clin Endocrinol Metab* 2010;95(2):707–713.
19. Kawasaki E. ZnT8 and type 1 diabetes. *Endocr J* 2012;59(7):531–537.
20. Davidson HW, Wenzlau JM, O'Brien RM. Zinc transporter 8 (ZnT8) and β cell function. *Trends Endocrinol Metab* 2014;25(8):415–424.
21. Shivaprasad C, Mittal R, Dharmalingam M, Kumar PK. Zinc transporter-8 autoantibodies can replace IA-2 autoantibodies as a serological marker for juvenile onset type 1 diabetes in India. *Indian J Endocrinol Metab* 2014;18(3):345–349.
22. Occhipinti M, Lampasona V, Vistoli F, Bazzigaluppi E, Scavini M, Boggi U et al. Zinc Transporter 8 Autoantibodies Increase the Predictive Value of Islet Autoantibodies for Function Loss of Technically Successful Solitary Pancreas Transplant. *Transplantation* 2011;92(6):674–677.
23. Rahbar S. An abnormal hemoglobin in red cells of diabetics. *Clin Chim Acta* 1968;22(2):296–298.
24. Peterson KP, Pavlovich JG, Goldstein D, Little R, England J, Peterson CM. What is hemoglobin A1c? An analysis of glycated hemoglobins by electrospray ionization mass spectrometry. *Clin Chem* 1998;44(9):1951–1958.

25. Bloomgarden ZT. A1C: Recommendations, debates, and questions. *Diabetes Care* 2009;32(12):e141–e147.
26. Incani M, Sentinelli F, Perra L, Pani MG, Porcu M, Lenzi A et al. Glycated hemoglobin for the diagnosis of diabetes and prediabetes: Diagnostic impact on obese and lean subjects, and phenotypic characterization. *J Diabetes Investig* 2015;6(1):44–50.
27. Selvin E, Steffes MW, Zhu H, Matsushita K, Wagenknecht L, Pankow J et al. Glycated hemoglobin, diabetes, and cardiovascular risk in nondiabetic adults. *N Engl J Med* 2010;362(9):800–811.
28. Selvin E, Ning Y, Steffes MW, Bash LD, Klein R, Wong TY et al. Glycated hemoglobin and the risk of kidney disease and retinopathy in adults with and without diabetes. *Diabetes* 2011;60(1):298–305.
29. Sacks DB. Measurement of hemoglobin A1cA new twist on the path to harmony. *Diabetes Care* 2012;35(12):2674–2680.
30. Radin MS. Pitfalls in hemoglobin A1c measurement: When results may be misleading. *J Gen Intern Med* 2013;29(2):388–394.
31. Freitas PAC, Ehlert LR, Camargo JL. Glycated albumin: A potential biomarker in diabetes. *Arch Endocrinol Metab* 2017;61(3):296–304.
32. Park S, Lee W, Chung HS, Hong KS. Diagnostic utility of serum glycated albumin for diabetes mellitus and its correlation with hyperlipidemia. *Ann Lab Med* 2016;36(4):306–312.
33. Hoshino J, Hamano T, Abe M, Hasegawa T, Wada A, Ubara Y et al. Glycated albumin versus hemoglobin A1c and mortality in diabetic hemodialysis patients: A cohort study. *Nephrol Dial Transplant* 2018;33(7):1150–1158.
34. Norimatsu K, Miura S, Suematsu Y, Shiga Y, Miyase Y, nakamura A et al. Associations between glycated albumin or hemoglobin A1c and the presence of coronary artery disease. *J Cardiol* 2015;65(6):487–493.
35. Buse JB, Freeman JL, Edelman SV, Jovanovic L, McGill JB. Serum 1,5-anhydroglucitol (GlycoMark): A short-term glycemic marker. *Diabetes Technol Ther* 2003;5(3):355–363.
36. Dungan KM, Buse JB, Largay J, Kelly MM, Button EA, Kato S et al. 1,5-Anhydroglucitol and postprandial hyperglycemia as measured by continuous glucose monitoring system in moderately controlled patients with diabetes. *Diabetes Care* 2006;29(6):1214–1219.
37. Pal A, Farmer AJ, Dudley C, Selwood MP, Barrow BA, Klyne R et al. Evaluation of serum 1,5 anhydroglucitol levels as a clinical test to differentiate subtypes of diabetes. *Diabetes Care* 2010;33(2):252–257.
38. Selvin E, Rawling AM, Grams M, Klein R, Steffes M, Coresh J. Association of 1,5-anhydroglucitol with diabetes and microvascular conditions. *Clin Chem* 2014;60(11):1409–1418.
39. Sato T, Kameyama T, Inoue H. Association of reduced levels of serum 1,5-Anhydro-d-glucitol with carotid atherosclerosis in patients with type 2 diabetes. *J Diabetes Complications* 2014;28(3):348–352.
40. Ikeda N, Hara H, Hiroi Y. 1,5-Anhydro-D-glucitol predicts coronary artery disease prevalence and complexity. *J Cardiol* 2014;64(4):297–301.
41. Ikeda N, Hara H, Hiroi Y, Nakamura M. Impact of serum 1,5-anhydro-d-glucitol level on prediction of major adverse cardiac and cerebrovascular events in non-diabetic patients without coronary artery disease. *Atherosclerosis* 2016;253:1–6.
42. Fujiwara T, Yoshida M, Akashi N, Yamada H, Tsukui T, Nakamura T et al. Lower 1,5-anhydroglucitol is associated with adverse clinical events after percutaneous coronary intervention. *Heart Vessels* 2016;31(6):855–862.

43. Ouchi S, Shimada K, Miyazaki T, Takahashi S, Sugita Y, Shimizu M et al. Low 1,5-anhydroglucitol levels are associated with long-term cardiac mortality in acute coronary syndrome patients with hemoglobin A1c levels less than 7.0. *Cardiovasc Diabetol* 2017;16(1):151.
44. de Oliveira EP, Burini RC. High plasma uric acid concentration: Causes and consequences. *Diabetol Metab Syndr* 2012;4:12.
45. Dehghan A, van Hoek M, Sijbrands EJ, Hofman A, Witteman JC. High serum uric acid as a novel risk factor for type 2 diabetes. *Diabetes Care* 2008;31(2):361–362.
46. Wang JY, Chen YL, Hsu CH, Tang SH, Wu CZ, Pei D. Predictive value of serum uric acid levels for the diagnosis of metabolic syndrome in adolescents. *J Pediatr* 2012;161(4):753-6.e2.
47. Bonakdaran S, Kharaqani B. Association of serum uric acid and metabolic syndrome in type 2 diabetes. *Curr Diabetes Rev* 2014;10(2):113–117.
48. Johnson RJ, Merriman T, Lanaspa MA. Causal or noncausal relationship of uric acid with diabetes. *Diabetes* 2015;64(8):2720–2722.
49. Simic MG, Jovanovic SV. Antioxidant mechanisms of uric acid. *J Am Chem Soc* 1989;111(15):5778–5782.
50. Sautin YY, Johnson RJ. Uric acid: The oxidant-antioxidant paradox. *Nucleosides Nucleotides Nucleic Acids* 2008;27(6):608–619.
51. Oda M, Satta Y, Takenaka O, Takahata N. Loss of urate oxidase activity in hominoids and its evolutionary implications. *Mol Biol Evol* 2002;19(5):640–653.
52. Lin SD, Tsai DH, Hsu SR. Association between serum uric acid level and components of the metabolic syndrome. *J Chin Med Assoc* 2006;69(11):512–516.
53. Yoo TW, Sung KC, Shin HS, Kim BJ, Kim BS, Kang JH, et al. Relationship between serum uric acid concentration and insulin resistance and metabolic syndrome. *Circ J* 2005;69(8):928–933.
54. Muraoka S, Miura T. Inhibition by uric acid of free radicals that damage biological molecules. *Pharmacol Toxicol* 2003;93(6):284–289.
55. Gill A, Kukreja S, Malhotra N, Chhabra N. Correlation of serum insulin and serum uric acid with glycated hemoglobin levels in patients of type 2 diabetes mellitus. *J Clin Diagn Res* 2013;7(7):1295–1297.
56. Rocic B, Lovrencic LV, Poje N, Poje M, Bertuzzi F. Uric acid may inhibit glucose-induced insulin secretion via binding to an essential arginine residue in rat pancreatic B-cells. *Bioorg Med Chem Lett* 2005;15(4):1181–1184.
57. Ames BN, Cathcart R, Schwiers E, Hochstein P. Uric acid provides an antioxidant defense in humans against oxidant- and radical-caused aging and cancer: A hypothesis. *Proc Natl Acad Sci U S A* 1981;78(11):6858–6862.
58. Whiteman M, Ketsawatsakul U, Halliwell B. A reassessment of the peroxynitrite scavenging activity of uric acid. *Ann N Y Acad Sci* 2002;962:242–259.
59. Jia Z, Zhang X, Kang S, Wu Y. Serum uric acid Levels and Incidence of impaired fasting glucose and type 2 diabetes mellitus: A meta-analysis of cohort studies. *Diab Res Clin Pract* 2013;101(1):88–96.
60. Corti A, Marcucci F, Bachetti T. Circulating chromogranin A and its fragments as diagnostic and prognostic disease markers. *Eur J Physiol* 2018;470(1):199–210.
61. Broedbaek K, Hilsted L. Chromogranin A as biomarker in diabetes. *Biomark Med* 2016;10(11):1181–1189.
62. D'amico MA, Ghinassi B, Izzicupo P, Manzoli L, Di Baldassarre A. Biological function and clinical relevance of chromogranin A and derived peptides. *Endocr Connect* 2014;3(2):R45–R54.

63. Schmid GM, Meda P, Caille D, Wargent E, O'Dowd J, Hochstrasser DF et al. Inhibition of insulin secretion by betagranin, an N-terminal chromogranin A fragment. *J Biol Chem* 2007;282(17):12717–12724.
64. Stadinski BD, Delong T, Reisdorph N, Reisdorph R, Powell RL, Armstrong M et al. Chromogranin A is an autoantigen in type 1 diabetes. *Nat Immunol* 2010;11(3):225–231.
65. Gottlieb PA, Delong T, Baker RL, Fitzgerald-Miller L, Wagner R, Cook G et al. Chromogranin A is a T cell antigen in human type 1 diabetes. *J Autoimmun* 2014;50:38–41.
66. Gerrits EG, Smit AJ, Bilo HJG. AGEs, autofluorescence and renal function. *Nephrol Dial Transplant* 2009;24(3):710–713.
67. Monami M, Lamanna C, Gori F, Bartalucci F, Marchionni N, Mannucci E. Skin autofluorescence in type 2 diabetes: Beyond blood glucose. *Diabetes Res Clin Pract* 2008;79(1):56–60.
68. Cahn F, Burd J, Ignotz K, Mishra S. Measurement of lens autofluorescence can distinguish subjects with diabetes From those without. *J Diabetes Sci Technol* 2014;8(1):43–49.
69. Calvo-Maroto AM, Perez-Cambrodi RJ, Garcia-Lazaro S, Ferrer-Blasco T, Cerviño A. Ocular autofluorescence in diabetes mellitus. A review. *J Diabetes* 2016;8(5):619–628.
70. Pehlivanoğlu S, Acar N, Albayrak S, Karakaya M, Ofluoğlu A. The assessment of autofluorescence of the crystalline lens in diabetic patients and healthy controls: Can it be used as a screening test? *Clin Ophthalmol* 2018;12:1163–1170.

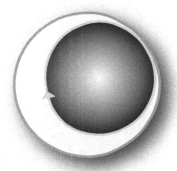

6 Anti-Diabetic Drugs

INTRODUCTION

The pharmacological treatments for diabetes differ for the type of diabetes, the plasma glucose and HbA1c criteria and the presence of diabetic complication(s). Although insulin was the first to be discovered among all anti-diabetic drugs, oral anti-diabetic drugs are the initiators for most types of diabetes except T1DM. Anti-diabetic drugs can be broadly classified into oral and parenteral. The oral drugs include classes such as biguanides, sulphonylureas, thiazolidinediones (TZDs), alpha-glucosidase inhibitors (AGIs), sodium glucose transporter-2 inhibitors (SGLT-2 inhibitors) and dipeptidyl peptidase-4 inhibitors (DPP-4 inhibitors), while the parenteral drugs include insulin, glucagon-like peptide-1 (GLP-1), analogues/mimetics and amylin analogue [1]. Whereas insulin is the mainstay for T1DM, the therapeutic approach for T2DM starts with oral anti-diabetic agents in which metformin is usually considered the first-line drug along with dietary precautions and lifestyle management. A combination of oral drugs is usually considered if the clinician, with their fine sense of judgement and analysis, feels it is the best approach to start with. Metformin is usually considered as one of the drugs in oral dual therapy too [1].Figure 6.1 shows various commercial anti-diabetic drug classes.

In the case of T1DM, whereby the insulin-producing beta-cells of the pancreas are destroyed as a result of autoimmune dysfunction, commercial insulin (administered as sub-cutaneous injection) still remains the mainstay of the therapeutic approach along with dietary precautions and lifestyle modifications. For T2DM patients, insulin is usually considered as the last tool when patients are not responding well to the oral anti-diabetics or the initial diagnosis is at a level where it is a must to initiate with insulin. As per the ADA, the starting dose of insulin is based on the body weight of the patient, whereby the initiating dose is 0.4–1.0 units/kg/day [2]. For the general knowledge of the readers, we must mention here that 1 unit of insulin is equivalent to 0.0347 mg of human insulin, as defined by the WHO Expert Committee on Biological Standardization [3]. The ADA and the Juvenile Diabetes Research Foundation (JDRF) also suggest that the initial dose could be 0.5 units/kg/day in metabolically active T1DM patients but the dose should be increased and adjusted if ketoacidosis is present [2]. Here, we must provide a very brief overview of the basic mechanism, types and dosage of recombinant insulin formulations present commercially. Insulin, as we all know, is a peptide hormone that maintains the level of blood glucose. It does this by transporting glucose from blood to the cells which convert and store glucose for other metabolic activities. The human cells which are sensitive to insulin-mediated glucose transport are adipocytes (fat cells), skeletal muscles and hepatocytes (liver cells). The glucose gets converted to fat or triglyceride in

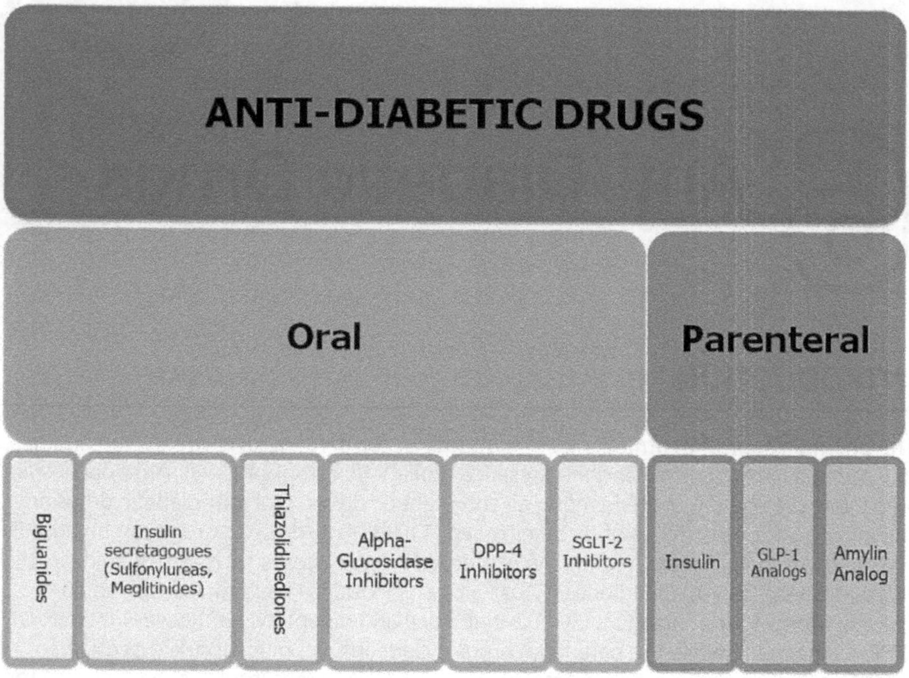

Figure 6.1 The commercial anti-diabetic drug classes.

adipocytes, and as glycogen in skeletal muscle cells and hepatocytes. The glucose enters these cells through a transmembrane glucose transporter known as GLUT-4. Before the invention and use of recombinant insulin, neutral protamine hagderon (NPH) insulin (animal protamine added to crude pig insulin) was used in patients but this preparation resulted in nocturnal hypoglycaemia that could lead to a potentially dangerous situation.

PARENTERAL ANTI-DIABETIC DRUGS (INSULIN)

The first recombinant human insulin was made by the pharmaceutical giant Eli Lilly in 1982, and was named Humulin®, with Humulin R as the short-acting and Humulin N as the intermediate-acting formulations. Now as per the physiological action, the insulin secretion is classified into basal and bolus. The small continuous insulin secretion throughout the day is known as basal, while the insulin amount released during or after a meal is known as bolus. Therefore, the recombinant human insulin was prepared and formulated in a way that it could provide glucose management throughout the day in a basal–bolus way [1]. Therefore, according to the action pattern, the commercial insulin formulations are available as bolus, prandial and pre-mixed. Secondly, commercial insulin is either human insulin or insulin analogues as per their structure. Insulin analogues are the insulin molecules that have a slight structural variation, mostly in terms of change of amino acid residue(s) or change in their position or both. In terms of their duration of action, insulin formulations are classified as rapid acting (action starts 15 minutes after administration), short acting (action starts 30 minutes after injection), intermediate acting (reaches systemic circulation 2–4 hours after administration), long acting (action starts over 24 hours) and ultra-long acting (action starts for up to 40 hours). Insulin glulisine (Apidra®), insulin lispro (Humalog®) and insulin aspart (Novolog®) are a few of the popular commercial rapid-acting analogues. Short-acting analogues include Humulin R and Novolin R. Humulin N and Novolin N are the popular intermediate-acting insulin analogues, while insulin detemir (Levemir®) and insulin glargine (Lantus) are the most popular commercial long-acting insulin analogues. Currently, insulin degludec is the only commercially available ultra-long acting insulin analogue. Pre-mixed insulin formulations available are 70/30 Humulin or Novolin (70% NPH insulin and 30% regular insulin), 50/50 Humulin (50% NPH insulin and 50% regular), 75/25 Humalog (75% protamine lispro and 25% lispro), 50/50 Humalog (50% protamine lispro and 50% lispro), 70/30 Novolog Neutral (70% protamine aspart and 30% aspart) and Ryzodeg 70/30 (70% degludec and 30% aspart). The pre-mixed formulations are basically a mixture of basal and prandial insulin/analogues and are considered better and safer as they reduce the mixing of insulin by the patients which may increase the chance of error. They are also better in mimicking the physiological basal–bolus insulin action. They are more convenient and are aimed at reducing the number of insulin injections per day [1, 4]. More details about insulin and analogues can be found in the References section (reference 1 and reference 4).

Apart from the conventional parenteral form of insulin available, the Mannkind Corporation has recently launched an inhaled insulin preparation named Afrezza®. It is a rapid-acting insulin formulation that needs to be taken at mealtimes. The inhaled formulation has several advantages as compared to the parenteral injectable insulin formulations. The first major advantage is patient compliance as regards the reduced need for painful injections. Secondly, it is much easier to carry while travelling as compared to insulin injections. Not forgetting the pharmacokinetic properties, Afrezza enters systemic circulation within 12 minutes and thus can quickly lower the elevated blood sugar. The peak effect is seen at 35 to 45 minutes after dosing. Afrezza comes in three dosage cartridges – 4 units, 8 units and 12 units. The most serious adverse event with Afrezza is possible severe bronchospasm in patients with chronic pulmonary disorders. As with other parenteral insulin formulations, hypoglycaemia still remains a serious adverse event with Afrezza. Other observed possible adverse events include a decline in pulmonary function, diabetic ketoacidosis and hyperkalaemia [5, 6].

Another parenteral anti-diabetic drug, Amylin analogue, is covered in the latter part of this chapter. As amylin analogue is not very commonly prescribed, the authors have mentioned it separately after oral anti-diabetic drugs.

There are drugs that are directly associated to the incretin system, such as GLP-1 agonists and DPP-4 inhibitors. Incretins are the hormones that are released on carbohydrate or fat consumption. They are released from the inner lining of the small intestine. The incretins stimulate initial insulin release long before the glucose flux is sensed by the pancreas islets. Thus, this augmentation of insulin release from the gut hormones has been termed as the 'incretin effect'. GLP-1 has also been shown to inhibit the glucagon secretion that is considered to be a great help to diabetic patients as diabetic patients with insulin resistance display hyperglucagonaemia, which is a major contributor to hyperglycaemia. The first GLP-1 analogue/agonist was Exenatide, which was a synthetic version of a peptide Exendin-4 isolated from the saliva of a reptile Gila monster (heloderma suspectum). Apart from Exenatide, several GLP-1 agonists have been approved recently such as liraglutide (Victoza; Novo Nordisk), albiglutide (Tanzeum; GSK), dulaglutide (Trulicity; Eli Lilly) and semaglutide (Ozempic; Novo Nordisk) [8–14]. Victoza is available in 1.2 mg and 1.8 mg once daily injections; Trulicity is available in 0.75 mg/0.5 ml and 1.5 mg/0.5 ml once weekly injections; and Ozempic is available in 0.5 mg/1 mg once weekly injections. GLP-1 agonists/analogues have been associated with pancreatitis, renal problems and skin hypersensitivity according to various reports and should be prescribed cautiously. GLP-1 agonists have a special warning about the possibility of thyroid tumour/ cancer. These drugs, therefore, should be monitored very carefully. Tanzeum was discontinued as of July 2018 [12].

ORAL ANTI-DIABETIC DRUGS

Oral anti-diabetic drugs are, in most cases, the mainstay of diabetes treatment until the physician diagnoses the need to start parenteral drugs (insulin, amylin and GLP-1 analogues). The initial anti-diabetic drugs were from a class of molecules known as sulphonylurea and biguanide. Sulphonylureas stimulate insulin secretion (insulin secretagogues), while biguanide increases insulin sensitivity in the insulin-responsive cells and also inhibits the extra hepatic gluconeogenesis. Sulphonylureas primarily bind to the SUR1 receptor on the β-cell membrane that follows the closure of ATP-K+ channels. This closure stimulates the opening of voltage-gates Ca^{2+} channels which results in the fusion of insulin granules with the membrane, and thus, their release into the blood. As this effect does not depend upon the plasma glucose concentration, sulphonylureas are, therefore, associated with an increased risk of hypoglycaemia. Another class of insulin secretagogues is from the meglitinide class (glinide class of drugs) which includes drugs such as repaglinide, mitiglinide and nateglinide. They bind to a separate receptor site compared to the conventional sulphonylureas, but they also stimulate insulin release in a similar manner that begins with closure of ATP-potassium channels [1, 4, 7]. Metformin, on the other hand, increases the peripheral insulin sensitivity in the skeletal muscles cells by stimulating the translocation of GLUT-1 receptors on the cell surface. Metformin was also reported to increase the endogenous secretion of GLP-1, thus improving further insulin responsiveness. Metformin, with minimum adverse effects as compared to all other anti-diabetic drugs, can be said to be the 'safest', and is considered to be the first-line therapy in diabetes. In terms of adverse effects, metformin is contraindicated in diabetic patients with severe renal damage as metformin can result in a life-threatening condition called lactic acidosis in such patients.

Estimated glomerular filtration rate (eGFR) is essential to determine before prescribing metformin. It has been reported that metformin is safe in patients with an eGFR >60 ml/min/1.73m². Dose adjustment with periodic eGFR check-up is recommended if eGFR is between 45–60 ml/min/1.73m². It is contraindicated in patients with eGFR <30 ml/min/1.73m². The FDA also states that metformin can be prescribed safely in diabetic patients with mild-to-moderate renal impairment, but the drug dosage should be adjusted based on periodic check-ups. It has also been reported that long-term metformin therapy can cause a deficiency of vitamin B_{12} in a few patients [1, 4, 8, 9]. Another oral drug class for diabetes that was initially controversial due to its cardiac and hepatic adverse effects is thiazolidinediones (glitazones or TZDs class of drugs). They are peroxisome proliferator-activated receptor-γ (PPAR-γ) agonists and activate the receptor on skeletal muscle cells and adipocytes. This activation results in increased glucose utilisation by these cells. Apart from this primary effect, TZDs also reduce hepatic glucose production. TZDs are also reported to remodel the adipocytes into small adipocytes that are more sensitive towards insulin as compared to the older cells. They have a prominent effect on triglyceride metabolism and reduce the free fatty acid (FFA) burden from the systemic circulation; thus, attenuating the insulin-resistant condition too. Due to this effect on FFA-insulin resistance pathways, TZDs are also important agents in obesity-induced diabetes where FFA-induced insulin resistance is a frequent event. Despite these beneficial effects, the use of TZDs has been limited due to their potential adverse events that are primarily cardiac, renal and hepatic. The two TZDs, rosiglitazones and pioglitazones, have been associated with peripheral water retention (oedema) and heart failure (oedema-related heart failure very commonly seen). This water retention is mainly caused due to the activation of the sodium channel in the distal nephron by this drug class. TZDs are also associated with decreased bone density, leading to increased fracture risk. Thus, TZDs should be cautiously prescribed in patients after effectively analysing the risk-to-benefit ratio [1, 4].

Alpha-glucosidase inhibitors (AGIs) are another class of anti-diabetic drugs that are considered comparatively safe. This class include drugs such as Acarbose, Miglitol and Voglibose. AGIs, as the name suggests, inhibit the alpha-glucosidase enzyme at the brush border of the small intestines, thus reducing the absorption of carbohydrates from the gut. This results in a decrease in blood glucose level. The major positive aspect is that these drugs do not cause hypoglycaemia, but major adverse effects include abdominal pain, flatulence and bloating. AGIs are very effective in decreasing the post-prandial glucose level and also the glycated haemoglobin (HbA1c) level. Other positive effects of AGIs include decreased lipid levels, improved GLUT-4-based glucose uptake and GLP-1 stimulation that in turn improves insulin sensitivity and action [1, 4].

Another 'incretin'-based therapy includes the DPP-4 inhibitors or the 'gliptin' class of drugs, which are oral anti-diabetic medications. DPP-4 is an enzyme present as a transmembrane protein that acts upon the endogenous incretins such as GLP-1 and degrades them. It is due to this enzyme that the half-life of endogenous GLP-1 is almost 5 minutes, which is pharmacologically much less. Thus, inhibition of DPP-4 results in the natural action of endogenous GLP-1 which enhances the insulin secretion. Sitagliptin (Januvia; Merck) was the first drug in this class to be approved by the US FDA in 2006, followed by vildagliptin (Galvus; Novartis) in 2007 [1, 15]. Other DPP-4 inhibitors are saxagliptin (Onglyza; AstraZeneca), alogliptin (Nesina; Takeda Pharmaceuticals), linagliptin (Tradjenta; Eli Lilly), trelagliptin (Zafatek; Takeda Pharmaceuticals) and teneligliptin (Tenelia; Daiichi Sankyo). The dosage regimens of these DPP-4 inhibitors are as follows: Sitagliptin (25/50/100 mg once daily), saxagliptin (2.5/5 mg once daily), vildagliptin (50/100 mg per day, not exceeding 100 mg daily), alogliptin (25 mg once daily), linagliptin (5 mg once daily), trelagliptin (100 mg once weekly) and teneligliptin (20 mg once daily). These DPP-4 inhibitors have been used as monotherapy or in combination with metformin, sulphonylureas, TZDs and insulin [16–23]. According to various studies and reports, the major adverse effects associated with DPP-4 inhibitors are pancreatitis, renal problems and even heart failure, which have also been put on the FDA warning list [24]. Therefore, these drugs should be used very cautiously in patients.

Another most recent addition to the list of oral anti-diabetic medicines is a class of drugs known as sodium-glucose co-transporter-2 inhibitors (SGLT-2 inhibitors or the 'gliflozin' drug class). These drugs inhibit a member SGLT-2 from a class of cell surface receptors found in the gastrointestinal tract and kidneys. This receptor is responsible for the passive transport of glucose and other monosaccharides. SGLT-2 receptors are primarily found in proximal renal tubules and are highly responsible for renal glucose reabsorption. It was also reported that the expression of SGLT-2 is significantly increased in diabetic patients. Thus, inhibiting these receptors would enhance renal glucose clearance by blocking glucose reabsorption, which raises the plasma glucose concentration. Canagliflozin (Invokana) was the first SGLT-2 inhibitor approved for use [1, 4]. It is also the only drug in this class that inhibits SGLT-1 receptors primarily present in the small intestine. Other drugs in this class include dapagliflozin (Forxiga), tofogliflozin (Deberza), empagliflozin (Jardiance), ipragliflozin (Suglat), luseogliflozin (Lusefi) and ertugliflozin (Steglatro). Invokana exists as a 300 mg tablet taken once daily; Forxiga exists as 5 mg and 10 mg tablets and the recommended dose is no more than 10 mg taken once daily; Jardiance comes as 10 mg and 25 mg pills taken once daily; Suglat comes in 25 mg and 50 mg tablets with the maximum dose not exceeding 100 mg per day; Lucefi exists in 2.5 mg and 5 mg pill formulations taken once daily; Steglatro, the latest addition to the class, is available in 5 mg and 15 mg formulations [25–31]. Regarding safety concerns and adverse events, SGLT-2 inhibitors have been shown to be associated with an increased risk of leg and foot amputation, diabetic ketoacidosis, urinary tract yeast infection, vaginal and penile yeast infection, bone fracture (by decreasing bone mineral density) and renal impairment [25–37]. These medications, therefore, should be very cautiously prescribed, taking into account the risk-to-benefit ratio. In a recently published large phase 3 multicentric trial (at 133 centres) evaluating the safety and efficacy of a new oral SGLT-2 inhibitor Sotagliflozin in combination with insulin in T1DM subjects, it was found that patients who received insulin along with Sotagliflozin had better reduction of HbA1c (below 7% recommended baseline value) as compared to the group taking insulin with a placebo. But the rate of ketoacidosis and hypoglycaemia was much higher in the treatment group than the placebo group. Thus, the concomitant use of SGLT-2 inhibitors with insulin should be prescribed with caution and proper monitoring [38].

Another supportive action for diabetes treatment comes from the hormone amylin, which is co-secreted along with insulin from the β-cells under glucose stimulus. Amylin, also known as islet amyloid polypeptide (IAPP), is a 37 amino acid residue long peptide that shares a similar promoter region with insulin. It has been reported that apart from glucose stimulus, amylin is also secreted well in response to arginine and fatty acids. The fasting state plasma amylin level is 3–5 pM, while the post-prandial value is 15–25 pM. Amylin primarily reduces glucose flux by delaying gastric emptying (thus slower glucose release in systemic circulation) and inhibiting glucagon secretion. In addition, it also reduces food intake as an action mediated by its interplay with the satiety centre in the central nervous system [39, 40]. Pramlintide (Symlin; AstraZeneca) is the first amylin analogue to be approved for use in diabetes in 2005. Pramlintide is structurally very similar to the endogenous amylin, created by replacing amino acid alanine at the 25th position and serine at the 28th and 29th positions by proline. Broadly, Pramlintide exerts its anti-hyperglycaemic action in two ways: It delays the gastric emptying of food and thus glucose release is slower. Secondly, it inhibits post-prandial glucagon secretion, which also reduces hepatic glucose production. Pramlintide is formulated as a subcutaneous injection and its bioavailability is almost 30–40%. The half-life of Symlin is approximately 48 minutes. Symlin is used along with insulin and never alone in the treatment of diabetes. Administration of Symlin usually reduces the dose of insulin by half in T2DM patients. Symlin is usually initiated with a dose of 60 mcg just before a meal in T2DM patients and that can be increased to 120 mcg as and when required and advised by a physician. In T1DM patients, the starting dose of Symlin should be 15 mcg. The dose can be further increased to 30 mcg, 45 mcg and 60 mcg as and when required and advised by the physician. The dose of Symlin is lesser in T1DM patients for the obvious fact of minimising the risk of hypoglycaemia, which could be serious for a patient with T1DM. The major adverse effect of Pramlintide is hypoglycaemia (not caused alone), and thus, the patient and their caretakers should watch closely for the related symptoms. Other minor adverse effects are nausea, abdominal pain, decreased appetite and indigestion. Injection site morbidity and bruising are common with almost all regular injectables. Symlin should not be used in patients who have confirmed gastroparesis and who are unaware of their hypoglycaemic events. Administration of Symlin along with insulin has shown to be effective in controlling glucose increment and effectively reduces HbA1c [40, 41]. Davalintide is a second-generation amylin analogue developed by Amylin Pharmaceuticals (now owned by AstraZeneca) that has shown great promise in delayed gastric emptying, inhibited glucagon secretion and reduction of food intake in animal models. Thus, it was also found to be very effective in lowering the plasma glucose [42]. Table 6.1 summarises various anti-diabetic drugs, their mode of action and related adverse events.

Table 6.1 Summary of Various Anti-Diabetic Drugs with Mechanism of Action and Adverse Events

Anti-Diabetic Drug Class (With One Example)	Mechanism of Action	Adverse Events
Biguanide (Metformin)	Inhibits hepatic gluconeogenesis, Increases insulin sensitivity, Increases GLUT-4 translocation	Rare case of lactic acidosis, Vitamin B_{12} deficiency
Sulphonylureas (Glimepiride)	Increases insulin secretion by binding to SUR1 receptors on -cells	Hypoglycaemia
Meglitinide (Repaglinide)	Increases insulin secretion by binding to -cells but the receptor is different than the sulphonylurea receptor	Lesser hypoglycaemic events as compared to sulphonylurea
α-glucosidase inhibitors (Voglibose)	Inhibit the α-glucosidase enzyme resulting in reduced carbohydrate absorption	Bloating, Diarrhoea
Thiazolidinediones (Pioglitazone)	PPAR-γ activators, Inhibit hepatic glucose production, Increase insulin sensitivity, Increase adiponectin level	Cardiovascular, renal and hepatic disorder, Peripheral oedema, Decreased bone mineral density
GLP-1 analogues (Exenatide)	Increase insulin secretion, Inhibit glucagon secretion	Pancreatitis, Renal disturbances and skin hypersensitivity
DPP-4 inhibitors (Sitagliptin)	Inhibit the DPP-4 enzyme resulting in prolonged action of endogenous GLP-1	Pancreatitis, Rare cases of heart failure
SGLT-2 inhibitors (Dapagliflozin)	Inhibit SGLT-2 receptors on the proximal renal tubules resulting in increased glycosuria	Increased risk of leg and foot amputation, Diabetic ketoacidosis, Urinary tract yeast infection, Vaginal and penile infection, Increased risk of bone fracture
Amylin analogues (Pramlintide)	Delayed gastric emptying thus slow glucose absorption, Inhibit glucagon secretion	Hypoglycaemia, if administered along with insulin, Decreased appetite, Nausea
Insulin	Acts on the insulin receptors resulting in increased glucose uptake through GLUT-4 receptors	Hypoglycaemia, Injection site morbidity

DRUGS FOR DIABETES INSIPIDUS

Synthetic AVP, known as desmopressin or DDAVP, is usually the drug of choice in DI patients, primarily central DI. DDAVP has an effective anti-diuretic effect with much less vasopressor action. Therefore, it does not increase local blood pressure. The drug can be given orally, intranasally or parentally. The half-life of the drug is 3.5 hours. The decrease in urine output, the primary target, will be observed in 1 to 2 hours of administration and the effect may remain anywhere between 6 and 18 hours. The oral daily dosage (approximately 20 times less potent than the intranasal formulation) varies from 100 to 1,200 µg in three divided doses, while the dosage for the intranasal formulation varies from 2 to 40 µg (once or twice a day). The parenteral dosage is usually 0.1 to 1 µg, usually once a day. The prostaglandin inhibitor such as Indomethacin acts by increasing the reabsorption of water and salts through proximal tubules in the kidneys. Indomethacin has become a treatment of choice in nephrogenic diabetes insipidus [43, 44]. Other drugs reported for the treatment of various forms of DI are Carbamazepine, Chlorpropamide, Clofibrate and thiazide diuretics.

DRUGS FROM THE LABS: THE STORY OF POSSIBILITIES

GK Activators

Glucokinase (GK), also known as hexokinase IV, is a glucose-phosphorylating enzyme expressed exclusively in the liver and β-cells that plays a crucial role in glucose homeostasis. It acts as a glucose-sensing enzyme in β-cells and plays a critical role in phosphorylating glucose to glucose-6-phosphate during glycolysis and glycogen synthesis in the liver. Apart from β-cells, they also play a role in glucose sensing in intestinal cells (enterocytes) and certain specialised neurons in the hypothalamus. Its effect is primarily induced in hepatocytes by insulin, while glucose acts as basic inducer of GK in β-cells. GK has a low affinity of glucose in the physiological range of 5 mmol/L to 7 mmol/L (90 mg/dL to 126 mg/dL) and it also lacks a feedback inhibition from its primary product glycose-6-phosphate (G6P). When the plasma glucose rises post-prandial, the β-cells sense this change and the uninterrupted influx of glucose into β-cells through GLUT2 leads to glucose fluctuation sensing and glucose-stimulated insulin secretion (GSIS). As the GK of β-cells, unlike other hexokinases, is not inhibited by G6P, its activity is essential in continuous sensing of glucose to stimulate GSIS. GK is said to exist in two different conformations, namely 'super open' and 'closed'. The super open conformation is the inactive form, while the closed conformation is the active state of GK. The conformation changes from super open to closed after glucose binding. Between super open and closed conformation, there is an intermediate 'open' confirmation. When the glucose binds to the super open form, the GK takes the closed structure. Upon binding of ATP, GK converts glucose to G6P. As soon as the G6P is released, the GK comes to the intermediate open form and binds another glucose molecule, if present. If glucose is not present, it gets back to the super open conformation. Thus, a continuous flux of glucose leads to a change of GK between closed and open, rather than closed and super open. In the liver, the action of GK is controlled by a protein known as glucokinase regulatory protein (GKRP). In low glucose condition (or high fructose-6-phosphate level), GKRP remains bound to GK, and sequesters it into the nucleus, rendering it inactive. As soon as the glucose level rises in the body (or there is an increase in fructose-1-phosphate), GKRP gets released and GK moves back to the cytoplasm and gets bound to glucose. This is essential to glycogenesis and glycolysis. In the low glucose state, the 'sensing' of GKRP in the liver prevents more glucose from getting converted to glycogen. As soon as the blood glucose rises, the glycogenesis starts again [45–47].

GK activation, because of its natural action, has long been thought of as a potential method to lower hyperglycaemia in diabetes patients. In animal models, it was shown that GK activators resulted in stimulated insulin secretion, reduced hepatic gluconeogenesis and improved glycaemic fluctuations. Though the initial GK activators significantly reduced blood glucose, most of them were withdrawn during phase 1 or 2 of the clinical trials due to three major problems incurred: They caused severe hypoglycaemia, they resulted in a significant elevation in plasma and liver triglyceride level, and thirdly they proved to be inactive in the long run. Hypoglycaemia resulted probably due to overstimulation of β-cell GK, while elevated plasma triglyceride was attributed to overstimulation of liver GK. The first major trial with a GK activator, MK-0941 developed by Merck & Co. (now withdrawn from the trial), revealed the increased incidences of hypoglycaemia and hypertriglyceridaemia with an increase in systolic blood pressure [48, 49]. As per the general targeting, GK activators have been divided into dual-targeting and liver-selective GK activators. Further, dual-targeting GK activators can be sub-classified into full GKA (increases the GK V_{max}; such as MK0941 and Dorzagliatin) and partial GKA (decreases Vmax; such as AZD1656 with withdrawn status) [50]. In a recent publication from Japan, researchers have synthesised the 'liver-specific' GK activator that would not cause a hypoglycaemic event due to activation of the β-cell GK enzyme and would not affect the liver and plasma triglyceride levels. TMG-123 from Teijin Pharma Ltd., Japan, is a liver-specific GK activator that has been tested in diabetes and obesity animal models [51]. The two currently active drugs in various phases of clinical trial are the molecule TTP399 (phase 2) from VTV Therapeutics, United States, and the second one is HMS5552 (Dorzagliatin; phase 2/3) developed by Hua Medicine, China. TTP399 is reported to be a liver-specific GK activator that does not affect the GK-GKRP interaction. The major positive points of TTP399 are that it does not increases the plasma/liver triglyceride, and does not result in diabetic ketoacidosis or hypoglycaemia, which were the two major adverse events with the earlier GK activators resulting in their withdrawal [52, 53]. Dorzagliatin, a dual-acting full GK activator is currently in a phase 3 trial (with metformin combination). Even as a combination medicine with metformin, it has shown no drug–drug interaction and is found to significantly improve the glycaemic parameters in T2DM patients [54]. Apart from the above two GK activators in clinical trials, there is a lot more research going into novel and potent GK activators. Two such trial reports, one of which is from China, that warrant a mention reveal promising anti-hyperglycaemic activity of a mangiferin (a glycosyl xanthone found in many plants such as mango bark and peel) as a potent GK activator both in *in vitro* and *in vivo* testing. In terms of plasma lipid status, the mangiferin reduced the plasma triglyceride, LDL, and HDL while it raised total cholesterol slightly in the treated diabetic group compared to the untreated diabetic group. Histological analysis reported a decrease in liver lipid deposition, which was a great observation as compared to the GK activators that were withdrawn for increase in liver and plasma lipids earlier in various clinical trials. Another major finding of the study was that mangiferin did not cause severe hypoglycaemia, which was observed in many GK activators [55]. In another recent report from Russia, conjoined structural derivatives containing two pyridoxine structures (pyridoxine dipharmacophore) were synthesised and displayed much better activation of glucokinase as compared to the test compound PF-04937319 (a GK activator candidate from Pfizer that was withdrawn in 2015 during clinical trials). Two of the compounds from the synthesised library, the most potent in the experiment, displayed very low toxicity in the animal model [56]. In another important discovery regarding GK activation, researchers from Japan have synthesised a thiophenyl-pyrrolidine derivative. The compound was found to be highly effective as a GK activator and produced minimum β-cell toxicity. It had significant blood glucose lowering activity in the animal model and was toxicologically very safe. The hypoglycaemia risk was also minimal, which is very important for GK activators [57]. In another encouraging report from Advinus Therapeutics, India, scientists synthesised a GK activator compound based on a 2-phenoxy-acetamide scaffold. The compound was predominantly liver specific with significant anti-hyperglycaemic activity but no hypoglycaemic events [58].

FGF21 Mimetics

Human fibroblast growth factor 21 (FGF21) is a 20 kDa protein hormone expressed primarily in the liver, white adipose tissue, pancreas and skeletal muscle cells. The action of FGF21 depends upon its binding to specific FGF receptors with a co-factor known as β-Klotho. This co-factor is predominantly expressed in the liver, pancreas and white adipose tissue. The FGF21 expression in the liver is controlled by PPAR-α, while its expression is controlled by PPAR-γ in adipocytes. The hormonal action of FGF21 in animals and humans is summarised to improve glucose homeostasis, lipid metabolism and preservation of β-cells. FGF21 stimulates the glucose uptake in mature adipocytes via GLUT1, which is an insulin-independent action. This leads to more triglyceride storage in adipocytes. On the other hand, FGF21 is shown to suppress hepatic glucose production, increase liver glycogen synthesis and lower glucagon production in mice models. It is also reported that the β-cell preserving action of FGF21 is mediated through Akt signalling pathways. Owing to these beneficial actions, the systemic administration of FGF21 protein has shown to reduce the plasma glucose in experimental rodents. Furthermore, FGF21 administration in monkeys resulted in significant lowering of FPG and fructosamine, while it increased the hepatic sensitivity of insulin in diabetic Wistar rat models. On the lipid profile front, systemic FGF21 administration resulted in significant reduction in plasma triglyceride, free fatty acids and total cholesterol in obese rodents and diabetic monkey models. On the obesity front, it is said to be an FGF21-resistant state as high circulating FGF21 has been found in obese rodents. FGF21 administration has also been shown to reverse hepatic steatosis. In human studies, it is shown that FGF21 plasma concentration is significantly increased in the insulin-resistant state and T2DM, but shows a decreasing trend in T1DM and LADA. FGF21 is shown to inversely correlate with muscle insulin sensitivity and have a direct correlation with the hepatic insulin resistance, FPG, 2-hour plasma glucose after an OGTT and HbA1c, reflecting a clear inter-relationship with the whole body and hepatic insulin resistance in T2DM in humans. Insulin-regulated FGF21 expression in skeletal muscle suggests that it is an insulin-dependent myokine. FGF21 has been shown to directly stimulate glucose uptake in skeletal muscles. The addition of mitiglinide, TZDs or subcutaneous insulin as an addition to metformin in T2DM subjects has shown to significantly reduce the circulating FGF21 levels in humans. This suggests that FGF21 decreases as the insulin sensitivity increases or that the metformin and TZDs related improved insulin sensitivity is attributed to a decreased FGF21. Hepatic expression of FGF21 and circulating FGF21 have been shown to be increased in fasting state possibly due to activation of PPAR-α by increased circulating free fatty acids and certain hormones (such as glucagon) that are stimulated in fasting state. The ketogenic diet (low carbohydrate and high fat) and low protein diet have been postulated to increase the production and circulation of FGF21. But as of yet, the role of FGF21 is still not well enough understood to decipher a cause–reason relationship with diabetes [59–61].Figure 6.2 summarises the action of FGF21 as reported in various literatures.

Owing to the various metabolic actions of FGF21, it has been seen as a potential drug candidate for diabetes and obesity. Several modified FGF21-based protein/peptides have been tested in various pre-clinical trials. PEGylated FGF21, recombinant Fc-FGF21, FGF21 mimetic antibodies and modified FGF21 have all undergone pre-clinical testing at different capacities at different locations globally. Though these FGF21 mimetics and modified FGF21 might not have been tested directly for diabetes, they have principal target actions against serious diabetes-related comorbidities. The prime mention goes to FGF21 mimetics LY-2405319 (by Eli Lilly) and PF-05231023 (also named CVX-343; developed by Pfizer). These two FGF21 mimetics, administered subcutaneously, displayed significant decrease in plasma triglyceride, LDL and total cholesterol, while there was an increase in HDL. But the glucose lowering effect was not markedly as great as what was observed in animal studies with these drugs. The adverse events were not serious, and the drugs were well tolerated. The not-so-great effect on blood glucose

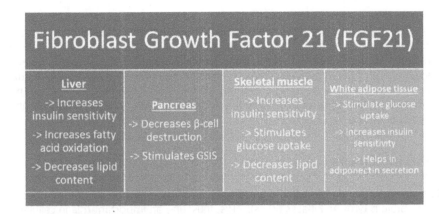

Fibroblast Growth Factor 21 (FGF21)

Liver	Pancreas	Skeletal muscle	White adipose tissue
-> Increases insulin sensitivity	-> Decreases β-cell destruction	-> Increases insulin sensitivity	-> Stimulate glucose uptake
-> Increases fatty acid oxidation	-> Stimulates GSIS	-> Stimulates glucose uptake	-> Increases insulin sensitivity
-> Decreases lipid content		-> Decreases lipid content	-> Helps in adiponectin secretion

Figure 6.2 Summarised actions of FGF21 in humans.

was possibly attributed to the metformin therapy the patients were on [59]. Though a few patients developed antibodies against LY-2405319, the effect was not neutralising and did not alter the pharmacokinetics of the drug. LY-2405319 was also related to improvement of insulin sensitivity and reduction in fasting hyperinsulinaemia [62]. In a recent publication by Talukdar et al. [63], a simultaneous pre-clinical (in monkeys) and clinical study for the effects of PF-05231023 was conducted. The drugs resulted in a significant reduction in body weight and triglyceride in the monkeys and obese T2DM humans, while adiponectin was elevated in both. IGF-1 increase was observed in humans. A significant increase in HDL was observed in test humans as compared to the control human subjects. But there was no significant reduction in plasma glucose and improvement in insulin sensitivity. One of the important adverse effects of this drug, though the exact mechanism has still not been deciphered, was a marked reduction in bone turnover and increased bone resorption. In another important development by Amgen Therapeutics, a modified Fc-FGF21 fusion protein was created (Fc-FGF21 RGE). It displayed great affinity towards the endogenous FGF21 receptor with increased half-life and reduced aggregation and degradation. The drug treatment in obese diabetic monkeys resulted in significant reduction in fasting plasma glucose, marked reduction in plasma triglyceride and significant increase in HDL. The test monkeys also significantly improved the oral glucose tolerance with significant reduction in fasting plasma insulin that showed an improvement in insulin sensitivity. There was also a significant reduction in body weight with an improvement in BMI [64]. In another recently published report, recombinant human FGF21 (rhFGF21) was administered subcutaneously to obese diabetic mice. The drug was shown to prevent β-cell destruction and resultant development of hyperglycaemia. It also improved oral glucose tolerance and clearance. It also resulted in browning of white adipose tissue, thus increasing energy expenditure. Surprisingly, the GLUT4 expression in white adipose tissue was observed to be increased, which resulted in insulin-stimulated glucose uptake [65]. In another very recent and exciting treatment option using FGF21, non-pathogenic adeno-associated virus (AAV) was used as a vehicle for FGF21 gene therapy mice model. This FGF21-containing vector was directed towards the liver, skeletal muscle and white adipose tissue. It enabled long-lasting (more than a year) maintenance of circulating FGF21 with a marked improvement in insulin sensitivity, reduction in body weight in obese animals and marked reduction in hepatic steatosis (also known as non-alcoholic steatohepatitis or NASH). It also resulted in the prevention of age-related weight gain and insulin resistance. There was a marked reversal of white adipose tissue hypertrophy and a significant increase in adiponectin level. As we know that adipose tissue inflammation is a hallmark of obesity, there was also a prevention of inflammation of white adipose tissue in the genetically treated animal models. The effect of the therapeutic intervention resulted in the circulating FGF21 and related therapeutic response for more than a year. This is perhaps the first FGF21-related gene therapy that resulted in a significant positive outcome and is definitely a ray of hope in diabetes and obesity treatment [66].

PTP-1B Inhibitors

Protein tyrosine phosphatases (PTPs) are the enzymes that have the diametrically opposite action to protein tyrosine kinases (PTKs). PTPs, thus, play an important role in cellular signalling processes by controlling the process of phosphorylation and dephosphorylation. The PTP family is classified into class I, II, III (cysteine-based enzymes) and IV (aspartate-based enzyme). Class I PTPs include phosphotyrosine-specific PTPs that are usually referred to as classical PTPs. These classical PTPs are either intracellular or transmembrane enzymes. PTP1B is a member of intracellular PTPs. It negatively regulates the insulin and leptin signalling in humans. PTP1B dephosphorylates the insulin receptor kinase that in turn downregulates the insulin signalling. Therefore, PTP1B inhibition is considered to be an important concept in the treatment of T2DM [67]. A few initial studies suggesting the inhibitory action of PTP1B on insulin signalling was reported in the early 1990s. Cicirelli et al. [68] reported that PTP-1B resulted in dephosphorylation of the insulin receptor, resulting in attenuation of insulin signalling. In another landmark study by Maegawa et al. [69], it was observed that high glucose concentration resulted in activation of PTP1B, which was responsible for attenuating the insulin signalling. Secondly, treatment with pioglitazone (a member of TZDs) resulted in a significant decrease in PTP1B that improved the insulin signalling. Elchebly et al. [70] demonstrated that mice lacking the PTP1B gene were more sensitive to insulin and they had a lesser concentration of circulating insulin that maintained the euglycaemic condition. Surprisingly, these mice were also resistant to obesity while on a high-fat diet. In order to gain a brief insight into insulin signalling, it is worth mentioning that insulin binds to its receptor, known as the insulin receptor. This receptor consists of two α-subunits (ligand binding) and two β-subunits (tyrosine kinase). When insulin binds to the α-subunits, the receptor gets autophosphorylated at various tyrosine residues due to the intrinsic kinase activity of the β-subunits. This autophosphorylation further leads to phosphorylation and activation of various downstream proteins, such as insulin receptor substrate (IRS). This IRS activation results in further PKB and PI-3 kinase activation. PKB activation results in translocation of GLUT-4 for glucose uptake and also induces indirect activation of glycogen synthase (active in dephosphorylated state) through deactivation of GSK-3 finally resulting in various biological actions of insulin. Activation of PKB and PI-3 kinase also inhibits hepatic gluconeogenesis. Various studies dating back over two decades found that PTP overactivity was involved in insulin resistance and diabetes [71, 72]. The original four classes of compounds viz. difluoromethylene phosphonates, 2-oxalylaminobenzoic acid, 2-carbomethoxybenzoic acid and a few other lipophilic compounds were identified to have a significant PTP1B inhibitory action. Since PTP1B interacts with epidermal growth factor (EGF), platelet-derived growth factor (PDGF) and insulin-like growth factor-1 (IGF-1), its inhibition might perturb this important signalling and therefore its usefulness as a drug target has been questionable [73]. It was also reported a decade ago that inflammatory factors such as TNF-α released from hypertrophied adipose tissues in obesity lead to overexpression of PTP1B which results in the attenuation of insulin signalling. The effect was very prominent with a high-fat diet. Therefore, pro-inflammatory cytokine, especially TNF-α, resulted in overexpression of PTP1B and disrupted the insulin signalling [74]. In another study involving polygenic diabetes mice models, PTP1B deficiency resulted in increased insulin and leptin sensitivity. Apart from the improvement in peripheral insulin sensitivity, PTP1B deficiency also resulted in the marked decrease in the hepatic gluconeogenic enzyme phosphoenolpyruvate carboxykinase. Hepatic phosphoenolpyruvate carboxykinase increased in the hepatic insulin-resistant case. Thus, a decrease in this enzyme indicated in improvement in hepatic insulin sensitivity [75]. Evidence regarding the role of PTP1B on pancreatic β-cells was recently provided by Ruiz et al. [76]. Silencing of PTP1B resulted in decreased apoptosis in β-cells from mice models. It also stabilised the streptozotocin-induced β-cell death in treated mice models. Moreover, the team also observed significant increase in glucose-stimulated insulin secretion in PTP1B silenced β-cells.

Regarding the various approaches to PTP1B inhibitor, as per the information available, only three drug candidates viz. Ertiprotafib, Trodusquemine and JTT-551, reached clinical trials (till phase 2) but were withdrawn due to various adverse effects. On the small molecule front, phosphotyrosine has been treated as the base scaffold to start the design of potent PTP1B inhibitors. Non-carboxylic acid derivatives were also designed and proved to be potent inhibitors of the enzyme. PTP1B inhibition was also sought out by using allosteric inhibitors. On the natural front, various terpenes and flavonoids from several natural sources demonstrated high PTP1B inhibitory potential [77]. The vast examples of such potential inhibitors and their design aspect can be read from the reference numbered 77. According to a very recent report, Ito et al. [78] developed an allosteric inhibitor KY-226 [4-(biphenyl-4-ylmethylsulphanylmethyl)-N-(hexane-1-sulphonyl)benzoylamide] against PTP1B. The molecule at the doses of 10 mg/kg/day and 30 mg/kg/day significantly decreased plasma glucose, triglyceride and HbA1c value in diabetic mice models without any increase in weight. The drug candidate also had marked anti-obesity effects on mice fed on a high-fat diet, owing to the leptin signal stimulation in the hypothalamus. Unlike the available drug Pioglitazone, the drug candidate KY-226 did not have any adverse effects, such as oedema and bone loss. The drugs, reported above, that reached clinical trial had PPARγ agonist activity too and resulted in adverse effects similar to that of TZDs. KY-226 did not exhibit such activity as it did not have any PPARγ agonist activity. In another report, a variety of TZD derivatives were designed and found to be highly potent PTP1B inhibitors. The glucose lowering effect (for the best of 36 compounds synthesised) was found to be better than that of the standard drug metformin [79]. In an effort to design an analogue of Trodusquemine, a team of researchers have synthesised DPM-1001, which is an orally bioactive PTP1B inhibitor. Both Trodusquemine (parent compound) and DPM-1001 are sterols but the former lacked oral bioavailability because it is a charged compound unlike DPM-1001 which is uncharged and had significant oral bioavailability [80]. Though Trodusquimine is a highly potent PTP1B inhibitor, its synthesis is quite labour- and cost-intensive with limited yield. Qin et al. reported in 2015 that synthesis of Claramine, an analogue of Trodusquimine, was easy to synthesise and has similar efficacy in inhibiting PTP1B. Claramine was equally effective in reducing blood glucose and decreasing body weight in obese diabetic animal models. Claramine was very effective in suppressing food intake by acting on the hypothalamus [81]. Among natural constituents, terpenoids, flavonoids, phenolic compounds, bromophenols, alkaloids and steroids have shown to potentially inhibit PTP1B. Maslinic acid (natural pentacyclic triterpene) derivatives, oleanolic acid derivatives, triterpene saponin derivatives, lithocholic acid derivatives and bromophenol derivatives have been reported to be highly potent PTP1B inhibitors [82]. Recently geranylated flavonoids from *Paulownia tomentosa* displayed significant PTP1B inhibition activity, also with additional α-glucosidase inhibition activity [83]. Recently, IONIS-PTP-1BRx, a second generation oligonucleotide antisense inhibitor of PTP1B, was highly effective in reducing blood glucose, HbA1c and leptin, and increasing the adiponectin level in a phase 2, double-blind, randomised, placebo-controlled, multicentre trial [84].

RAGE Inhibitors

As covered in Chapter 4, AGEs are the non-enzymatically generated glycated products as a result of persistent hyperglycaemia. AGEs are basically the modified form of physiological macromolecules. These modified macromolecules show altered functions that serve as the basis of dysfunctions. AGEs are reported to be responsible for various diabetes-related complications. The highly reactive carbonyl methylglyoxal is usually considered the primary precursor of AGE development. Receptors for AGE (RAGE) are a member of the immunoglobulin superfamily that upon interaction with AGE leads to cellular stress, damage and finally tissue/organ dysfunction. RAGE consists of a cytoplasmic domain and a charged transmembrane domain, while the extracellular domain consists of a V-type subdomain and two C-type subdomains. Apart from the AGEs, a wide variety of non-AGE ligands such as S100/calgranulins, HMGB1, lipopolysaccharides, β-amyloids and C1q binds to RAGEs. Such signallings are highly reflective of an inflammatory state. In atherosclerotic animal models, it has been reported that RAGEs are highly expressed on smooth muscle cells and macrophages and blocking RAGEs resulted in attenuation of accelerated atherosclerosis. Disruption of AGE–RAGE signalling has been widely studied through soluble RAGE (sRAGE). sRAGE is a truncated extracellular portion of RAGE that is detectable in blood. It has been reported that sequestration of various AGEs *in vivo* resulted in inhibition of interaction between AGEs and RAGEs, thus finding this concept therapeutically very effective. It has been verified in several experimental studies that blocking RAGE (even by using soluble RAGE) resulted in marked improvement in cases such as E. coli sepsis, pneumococcal pneumonia, influenza A-assisted pneumonia and diabetic periodontitis. Secondly, administration of sRAGE in diabetic mice models resulted in a significant decrease in the expression of inflammatory markers and RAGE in the pancreas. It was also reported that chronic treatment with sRAGE even for over 6 months in mice models resulted in no adverse events. Treatment with sRAGE also attenuated the diabetic retinopathy characteristics such as breakdown of blood-brain-barrier (BBB), leukostasis and lesion development [85, 86]. Some small-molecule-based AGE inhibitors have also been developed such as aminoguanidine, pyridoxamine and OPB-9195 [(±)–2-isopropylidenehydrazono-4-oxo-thiazolidin-5-ylac etanilide)], which are shown to significantly inhibit the AGE formation. Marketed drugs such as metformin and atorvastatin have even also shown to have a marked effect on decreasing AGE formation. N-phenacylthiazolium bromide

(PTB) and ALT-711 (Alagebrium) are two widely known experimental AGE breakers. Another potential drug molecule, Kremezin, was shown to markedly decrease the serum AGE levels in patients. Treatment with Kremezin also attenuated the expression of RAGEs, monocyte chemoattractant protein-1 (MCP-1) and vascular cell adhesion molecule-1 (VCAM-1) on the endothelial cells. Anti-hypertensives such as angiotensin-converting enzyme inhibitors (ACEIs) and angiotensin II receptor blockers (ARBs) decrease the formation of AGEs. Telmisartan was reported to decrease the expression of RAGEs and MCP-1 in the mesangial cells, while it also decreased the production of superoxide ions and other ROS [87]. Aminoguanidine traps the reactive carbonyl moieties, and thus prevents the formation of AGEs. But even today, there is no scientific evidence that aminoguanidine works for humans. Pyridoxamine, on the other hand, has been described to chelate Amadori products such as fructoselysine. It also blocks the oxidation of intermediates in the Amadori reaction and traps the highly reactive carbonyl and dicarbonyl compounds [88]. For those interested in the medicinal chemistry and drug designing aspect of RAGE inhibition, a wide range of compounds have been described in references 88 and 89.

REFERENCES

1. Kumar A, Bharti SK, Kumar A. Therapeutic molecules against type 2 diabetes: What we have and what are we expecting? *Pharmacol Rep* 2017;69(5):959–970.
2. American Diabetes Association. Pharmacologic approaches to glycemic treatment: Standards of medical care in diabetes-2018. *Diabetes Care* 2018;41(Suppl 1):S73–S85.
3. Accessed at www.who.int/biologicals/expert_committee/BS_2143_Human_Recombinant_Insulin_final.pdf; accessed on June 26, 2018.
4. Upadhyay J, Polyzos SA, Perakakis N, Thakkar B, Paschou SA, Katsiki N et al. Pharmacotherapy of type 2 diabetes: An update. *Metabolism* 2018;78:13–42.
5. Accessed at http://investors.mannkindcorp.com/news-releases/news-release-details/fda-updates-afrezzar-prescribing-information.
6. Accessed at www.accessdata.fda.gov/drugsatfda_docs/label/2014/022472lbl.pdf.
7. Massi-Benedetti M, Damsbo P. Pharmacology and clinical experience with repaglinide. *Expert Opin Investig Drugs* 2000;9(4):885–898.
8. Maruthur NM, Tseng E, Hutfless S, Wilson LM, Suarez-Cuervo C, Berger Z et al. Diabetes medications as monotherapy or metformin-based combination therapy for Type 2 diabetes: A systematic review and meta-analysis. *Ann Intern Med* 2016;164(11):740–751.
9. Accessed at www.fda.gov/downloads/Drugs/DrugSafety/UCM494140.pdf; accessed on August 14, 2018.
10. Holst JJ, Vilsbøll T, Deacon CF. The incretin system and its role in type 2 diabetes mellitus. *Mol Cell Endocrinol* 2009;297(1–2):127–136.
11. Accessed at www.victoza.com/; accessed on August 16, 2018.
12. Accessed at www.tanzeum.com/; accessed on August 16, 2018.
13. Accessed at www.trulicity.com/; accessed on August 16, 2018.
14. Accessed at www.ozempic.com/; accessed on August 16, 2018.
15. Karagiannis T, Boura P, Tsapas A. Safety of dipeptidyl peptidase 4 inhibitors: A perspective review. *Ther Adv Drug Saf* 2014;5(3):138–146.
16. Accessed at www.januvia.com/; accessed on August 17, 2018.
17. Accessed at www.ema.europa.eu/ema/index.jsp?curl=pages/medicines/human/medicines/000771/human_med_000803.jsp&mid=WC0b01ac058001d124; accessed on August 17, 2018.
18. Accessed at www.onglyza.com/; accessed on August 17, 2018.

19. Accessed at www.nesinafamily.com/; accessed on August 17, 2018.
20. Accessed at https://general.takedapharm.com/NESINAPI; accessed on August 17, 2018.
21. Accessed at www.tradjenta.com/; accessed on August 17, 2018.
22. Accessed at www.takeda.com/newsroom/newsreleases/2015/new-drug-applicati on-approval-of-zafatek-tablets-for-the-treatment-of-type-2-diabetes-in-japan/; accessed on August 17, 2018.
23. Accessed at www.daiichisankyo.com/media_investors/media_relations/press_relea ses/detail/006054.html; accessed on August 17, 2018.
24. Accessed at www.fda.gov/Drugs/DrugSafety/ucm486096.htm; accessed on August 17, 2018.
25. Accessed at www.invokana.com/about-invokana/what-is-invokana; accessed on August 18, 2018.
26. Accessed at www.astrazeneca.ca/content/dam/az-ca/downloads/productinform ation/forxiga-consumer-information-leaflet-en.pdf; accessed on August 18, 2018.
27. Accessed at www.ema.europa.eu/docs/en_GB/document_library/EPAR_-_Summary _for_the_public/human/002322/WC500136025.pdf; accessed on August 18, 2018.
28. Accessed at www.jardiance.com/; accessed on August 18, 2018.
29. Accessed at www.astellas.com/en/corporate/news/detail/approval-of-suglat-tablets -a-s.html; accessed on August 18, 2018.
30. Accessed at http://lusefi.jp/english/di.html#di04; accessed on August 18, 2018.
31. Accessed at www.steglatro.com/; accessed on August 18, 2018.
32. Accessed at www.fda.gov/Drugs/DrugSafety/ucm557507.htm; accessed on August 18, 2018.
33. Accessed at www.fda.gov/Drugs/DrugSafety/ucm505860.htm; accessed on August 18, 2018.
34. Accessed at www.fda.gov/Drugs/DrugSafety/ucm475463.htm; accessed on August 18, 2018.
35. Accessed at www.fda.gov/Drugs/DrugSafety/ucm461449.htm; accessed on August 18, 2018.
36. Accessed at www.merck.com/product/usa/pi_circulars/s/steglatro/steglatro_pi.pdf; accessed on August 18, 2018.
37. Accessed at www.merck.com/product/usa/pi_circulars/s/steglatro/steglatro_mg.pdf; accessed on August 18, 2018.
38. Garg SK, Henry RR, Banks P, Buse JB, Davies MJ, Fulcher GR et al. Effects of sotagliflozin added to insulin in patients with type 1 diabetes. *N Engl J Med* 2017;377(24):2337–2348.
39. Hay DL, Chen S, Lutz TA, Parkes DG, Roth JD. Amylin: Pharmacology, physiology, and clinical potential. *Pharmacol Rev* 2015;67(3):564–600.
40. Accessed at www.accessdata.fda.gov/drugsatfda_docs/label/2005/021332lbl.pdf; accessed on August 18, 2018.
41. Accessed at www.fda.gov/downloads/Drugs/DrugSafety/ucm089141.pdf; accessed on August 18, 2018.
42. Mack CM, Smith PA, Athanacio JR, Xu K, Wilson JK, Reynolds JM et al. Glucoregulatory effects and prolonged duration of action of davalintide: A novel amylinomimetic peptide. *Diab Obes Metab* 2011;13(12):1105–1113.
43. Di Iorgi N, Napoli F, Allegri AE, Olivieri I, Bertelli E, Gallizia A et al. Diabetes insipidus- -Diagnosis and management. *Horm Res Paediatr* 2012;77(2):69–84.
44. Bockenhauer D, Bichet DG. Pathophysiology, diagnosis and management of nephrogenic diabetes insipidus. *Nat Rev Nephrol* 2015;11(10):576–588.

45. Lenzen S. A fresh view of glycolysis and glucokinase regulation: History and current status. *J Biol Chem* 2014;289(18):12189–12194.
46. Baltrusch S, Tiedge M. Glucokinase regulatory network in pancreatic β-Cells and liver. *Diabetes* 2006;55(Suppl 2):S55–S64.
47. Iynedjian PB. Molecular physiology of mammalian glucokinase. *Cell Mol Life Sci* 2009;66(1):27–42.
48. Agius L. Lessons from glucokinase activators: The problem of declining efficacy. *Expert Opin Ther Pat* 2014;24(11):1155–1159.
49. Meininger GE, Scott R, Alba M, Shentu Y, Luo E, Amin H et al. Effects of MK-0941, a novel glucokinase activator, on glycemic control in insulin-treated patients with type 2 diabetes. *Diabetes Care* 2011;34(12):2560–2566.
50. Zhu XX, Zhu DL, Li XY, Li YL, Jin XW, Hu TX et al. Dorzagliatin (HMS5552), a novel dual-acting glucokinase activator, improves glycaemic control and pancreatic β-cell function in patients with type 2 diabetes: A 28-day treatment study using biomarker-guided patient selection. *Diabetes Obes Metab* 2018;20(9):2113–2120.
51. Tsumura Y, Tsushima Y, Tamura A, Hasebe M, Kanou M, Kato H et al. TMG-123, a novel glucokinase activator, exerts durable effects on hyperglycemia without increasing triglyceride in diabetic animal models. *PLoS One* 2017;12(2):e0172252.
52. Accessed at www.vtvtherapeutics.com/assets/docs/TTP399_ADA GKRP_05292015 _pdf.pdf.
53. Accessed at www.vtvtherapeutics.com/assets/ada_gka_poster_lb_june2018.pdf.
54. Chen L, Zhao G, Ren S, Zhang Y, Du D. No drug–drug interaction between dorzagliatin and metformin in type 2 diabetes patients. *Diabetes* 2018 Jul;67(Suppl 1). doi:10.2337/db18-2310-PUB.
55. Min Q, Cai X, Sun W, Gao F, Li Z, Zhang Q et al. Identification of mangiferin as a potential glucokinase activator by structure-based virtual ligand screening. *Sci Rep* 2017;7:44681.
56. Dzyurkevich MS, Babkov DA, Shtyrlin NV, Mayka OY, Iksanova AG, Vassiliev PM et al. Pyridoxine dipharmacophore derivatives as potent glucokinase activators for the treatment of type 2 diabetes mellitus. *Sci Rep* 2017;7(1):16072.
57. Fujieda H, Kogami M, Sakairi M, Kato N, Makino M, Takahashi N et al. Discovery of a potent glucokinase activator with a favorable liver and pancreas distribution pattern for the treatment of type 2 diabetes mellitus. *Eur J Med Chem* 2018;156:269–294.
58. Deshpande AM, Bhuniya D, De S, Dave B, Vyavahare VP, Kurhade SH et al. Discovery of liver-directed glucokinase activator having anti-hyperglycemic effect without hypoglycemia. *Eur J Med Chem* 2017;133:268–286.
59. So WY, Leung PS. Fibroblast growth factor 21 as an emerging therapeutic target for type 2 diabetes mellitus. *Med Res Rev* 2016;36(4):672–704.
60. Iglesias P, Selgas R, Romero S, Díez JJ. Biological role, clinical significance, and therapeutic possibilities of the recently discovered metabolic hormone fibroblastic growth factor 21. *Eur J Endocrinol* 2012;167(3):301–309.
61. Strowski MZ. Impact of FGF21 on glycemic control. *Horm Mol Biol Clin Investig* 2017;30(2). doi:10.1515/hmbci-2017-0001.
62. Reitman ML. FGF21 mimetic shows therapeutic promise. *Cell Metab* 2013;18(3):307–309.
63. Talukdar S, Zhou Y, Li D, Rossulek M, Dong J, Somayaji V et al. A long-acting FGF21 molecule, PF-05231023, decreases body weight and improves lipid profile in non-human primates and type 2 diabetic subjects. *Cell Metab* 2016;23(3):427–440.
64. Stanislaus S, Hecht R, Yie J, Hager T, Hall M, Spahr C et al. A novel Fc-FGF21 with improved resistance to proteolysis, increased affinity toward β-klotho, and enhanced efficacy in mice and cynomolgus monkeys. *Endocrinology* 2017;158(5):1314–1327.

65. Laeger T, Baumeier C, Wilhelmi I, Würfel J, Kamitz A, Schürmann A. FGF21 improves glucose homeostasis in an obese diabetes-prone mouse model independent of body fat changes. *Diabetologia* 2017;60(11):2274–2284.
66. Jimenez V, Jambrina C, Casana E, Sacristan V, Muñoz S, Darriba S et al. FGF21 gene therapy as treatment for obesity and insulin resistance. *EMBO Mol Med* 2018;10(8):pii: e8791.
67. Tamrakar AK, Maurya CK, Rai AK. PTP1B inhibitors for type 2 diabetes treatment: A patent review (2011 - 2014). *Expert Opin Ther Pat* 2014;24(10):1101–1115.
68. Cicirelli MF, Tonks NK, Diltz CD, Weiel JE, Fischer EH, Krebs EG. Microinjection of a protein-tyrosine-phosphatase inhibits insulin action in Xenopus oocytes. *Proc Natl Acad Sci U S A* 1990;87(14):5514–5518.
69. Maegawa H, Ide R, Hasegawa M, Ugi S, Egawa K, Iwanishi M et al. Thiazolidine derivatives ameliorate high glucose-induced insulin resistance via the normalization of protein-tyrosine phosphatase activities. *J Biol Chem* 1995;270(13):7724–7730.
70. Elchebly M, Payette P, Michaliszyn E, Cromlish W, Collins S, Loy AL et al. Increased insulin sensitivity and obesity resistance in mice lacking the protein tyrosine phosphatase-1B gene. *Science* 1999;283(5407):1544–1548.
71. Kennedy BP. Role of protein tyrosine phosphatase-1B in diabetes and obesity. *Biomed Pharmacother* 1999;53(10):466–470.
72. Gum RJ, Gaede LL, Koterski SL, Heindel M, Clampit JE, Zinker BA et al. Reduction of protein tyrosine phosphatase 1B increases insulin-dependent signaling in ob/ob mice. *Diabetes* 2003;52(1):21–28.
73. Johnson TO, Ermolieff J, Jirousek MR. Protein tyrosine phosphatase 1B inhibitors for diabetes. *Nat Rev Drug Discov* 2002;1(9):696–709.
74. Zabolotny JM1, Kim YB, Welsh LA, Kershaw EE, Neel BG, Kahn BB. Protein-tyrosine phosphatase 1B expression is induced by inflammation in vivo. *J Biol Chem* 2008;283(21):14230–14241.
75. Xue B, Kim YB, Lee A, Toschi E, Bonner-Weir S, Kahn CR et al. Protein-tyrosine phosphatase 1B deficiency reduces insulin resistance and the diabetic phenotype in mice with polygenic insulin resistance. *J Biol Chem* 2007;282(33):23829–23840.
76. Fernandez-Ruiz R, Vieira E, Garcia-Roves PM, Gomis R. Protein tyrosine phosphatase-1B modulates pancreatic B-cell mass. *PLoS One* 2014;9(2):e90344.
77. Qian S, Zhang M, He Y, Wang W, Liu S. Recent advances in the development of protein tyrosine phosphatase 1B inhibitors for type 2 diabetes. *Future Med Chem* 2016;8(11):1239–1258.
78. Ito Y, Fukui M, Kanda M, Morishita K, Shoji Y, Kitao T et al. Therapeutic effects of the allosteric protein tyrosine phosphatase 1B inhibitor KY-226 on experimental diabetes and obesity via enhancements in insulin and leptin signaling in mice. *J Pharmacol Sci* 2018;137(1):38–46.
79. Liu Z, Chai Q, Li YY, Shen Q, Ma LP, Zhang LN et al. Discovery of novel PTP1B inhibitors with antihyperglycemic activity. *Acta Pharmacol Sin* 2010;31(8):1005–1012.
80. Krishnan N, Konidaris KF, Gasser G, Tonks NK. A potent, selective, and orally bioavailable inhibitor of the protein-tyrosine phosphatase PTP1B improves insulin and leptin signaling in animal models. *J Biol Chem* 2018;293(5):1517–1525.
81. Qin Z, Pandey NR, Zhou X, Stewart CA, Hari A, Huang H et al. Functional properties of Claramine: A novel PTP1B inhibitor and insulin-mimetic compound. *Biochem Biophys Res Commun* 2015;458(1):21–27.
82. Wang LJ, Jiang B, Wu N, Wang SY, Shi DY. Natural and semisynthetic protein tyrosinephosphatase 1B (PTP1B) inhibitors as anti-diabetic agents. *RSC Adv* 2015;5(60):48822.

83. Song YH, Uddin Z, Jin YM, Li Z, Curtis-Long MJ, Kim KD et al. Inhibition of protein tyrosine phosphatase (PTP1B) and α-glucosidase by geranylated flavonoids from Paulownia tomentosa. *J Enzyme Inhib Med Chem* 2017;32(1):1195–1202.
84. Digenio A, Pham NC, Watts LM, Morgan ES, Jung SW, Baker BF et al. Antisense inhibition of protein tyrosine phosphatase 1B With IONIS-PTP-1BRx improves insulin sensitivity and reduces weight in overweight patients with type 2 diabetes. *Diabetes Care* 2018;41(4):807–814.
85. Manigrasso MB, Juranek J, Ramasamy R, Schmidt AM. Unlocking the biology of RAGE in diabetic microvascular complications. *Trends Endocrinol Metab* 2014;25(1):15–22.
86. Ramasamy R, Yan SF, Schmidt AM. Receptor for AGE (RAGE): Signaling mechanisms in the pathogenesis of diabetes and its complications. *Ann N Y Acad Sci* 2011;1243:88–102.
87. Yamagishi S, Nakamura K, Matsui T, Ueda S, Noda Y, Imaizumi T. Inhibitors of advanced glycation end products (AGEs): Potential utility for the treatment of cardiovascular disease. *Cardiovasc Ther* 2008;26(1):50–58.
88. Nagai R, Murray DB, Metz TO, Baynes JW. Chelation: A fundamental mechanism of action of AGE inhibitors, AGE breakers, and other inhibitors of diabetes complications. *Diabetes* 2012;61(3):549–559.
89. Bongarzone S, Savickas V, Luzi F, Gee AD. Targeting the receptor for advanced glycation endproducts (RAGE): A medicinal chemistry perspective. *J Med Chem* 2017;60(17):7213–7232.

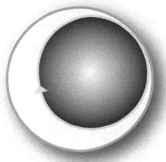

7 Diagnosis and Treatment

DIAGNOSIS OF DIABETES

Proper diagnosis of any disease is the first thing that should be done before medications can be initiated just on the basis of symptoms. Diabetes can very often be asymptomatic in its initial period, but as the disease progresses and starts affecting organs, gradual symptoms appear. The three cardinal signs of diabetes are polyuria (excessive urination), polydipsia (excessive thirst) and polyphagia (excessive hunger). These signs are quite common in T1DM but can be found in T2DM patients with prolonged uncontrolled hyperglycaemia [1, 2]. Other symptoms that may occur as a result of uncontrolled hyperglycaemia include numbness or pain in extremities (dysesthesia), ketoacidosis, vision problems, non-healing wounds, recurrent urogenital infections, dry mouth and acanthoses nigricans (dark patch present in arm pit, neck and groin area due to insulin resistance). Diabetic ketoacido sis (DKA) is common in T1DM but could be present in prolonged uncontrolled hyperglycaemic state in T2DM [1, 2]. Therefore, proper pathological diagnosis is critical in relating them with the above-mentioned symptoms to confirm the presence of diabetes.

The common diagnostic criteria for diabetes depend upon the measurement of blood glucose and a haemoglobin variant that is actually glycosylated haemoglobin (HbA1c). These criteria include fasting plasma glucose (FPG), a 2-hour plasma glucose test following a 75-gram glucose ingestion (oral glucose tolerance test or OGTT; 2-h PG) and HbA1c value. Apart from these three diagnoses that are common for both T1DM and T2DM, the former has certain unique diagnostic features due to its autoimmune nature. T1DM patients have certain unique autoantibodies, namely islet cell antibodies (ICA), glutamic acid decarboxylase antibody (GAD-65), insulin autoantibodies (IAA), insulinoma antigen-2 protein (IA-2; a tyrosine phosphatase) and zinc transporter 8 variant (ZnT8) antibody. It has been reported that almost 95% of T1DM patients express at least one of these autoantibodies. The most commonly prevalent autoantibody in the case of T1DM is GAD-65, which is reported to be present in almost 80% of diagnosed T1DM patients. T1DM patients very commonly have diagnosed diabetic ketoacidosis [2–5]. As per the glucose-based criteria, the following values are recommended by the American Diabetes Association (ADA), which formulates the global guidelines for diabetes [6]:

1) FPG ≥126 mg/dL (7 mmol/L) after at least 8 hours of fasting
2) 2-h PG ≥200 mg/dL (11.1 mmol/L); after consumption of 75 grams glucose solution
3) HbA1c ≥6.5% (48 mmol/mol)

Apart from these tests, a random glucose test (random plasma glucose or RPG) is also often performed and the plasma glucose value equal to or greater than 200 mg/

dL suggests a diabetic state. The ADA also suggests the presence of at least two autoantibodies for the confirmation of T1DM, although the antibody specificity and titre would denote the progression and stage of T1DM. But the glucose-dependent factors (FPG, HbA1c, OGTT and RPG) are raised long before the onset of the diabetic symptoms [6]. As a special instruction, to avoid misdiagnosis, the HbA1c should be measured as per the NGSP (National Glycohemoglobin Standardization Program) certified criteria and standardised to the DCCT (Diabetes Control and Complications Trial) assay points. The ADA recommends that the clinical diagnosis should be confirmed when at least two glucose-dependant criteria turn out to be positive (same test twice at different points in time or two different tests). But as a point of caution, the ADA also states that as compared to the FPG and HbA1c tests, the 2-h PG diagnoses more people with diabetes [6]. The Joslin Diabetes Centre also states that the point-of-care HbA1c testing may not be considered very reliable and should not be accepted for the diagnosis of diabetes [7]. Considering the accelerated cases of diabetes globally, the ADA and physicians recommend the testing of 'pre-diabetes' condition. Pre-diabetes is considered when the plasma glucose levels do not meet the diabetes criteria but are high enough to not be normal. Patients are diagnosed with an impaired fasting glucose (IFG), impaired glucose tolerance (IGT), and HbA1c level between 5.7–6.4%. IFG is defined as the plasma glucose value between 100–125 mg/dL, while IGT is considered to be a 2-h PG value between 140–199 mg/dL.

A third type of diabetes, known as gestational diabetes mellitus (GDM), is often considered as a temporary condition as most of the women recover from the hyperglycaemic condition post-delivery. As per the ADA, GDM is defined as the diabetic state that is diagnosed for the first time during the second or third trimester of the pregnancy and was not present before conception. If the diabetes diagnosis is made during the early pregnancy stage, it can be treated as pre-existing pre-gestational diabetes. Proper diagnosis and screening of GDM is essential as it can increase the chances of premature birth, foetal growth abnormalities, delivery issues, increased rate of caesarean section and development of diabetes in mother and infant post-delivery. The screening guidelines by the ADA suggest 2-hour 75-gram glucose OGTT. Three samples are considered with the first sample being the fasting sample, the second sample at 1 hour post-glucose consumption and the third sample 2 hours after the glucose consumption. GDM is confirmed when the plasma glucose for the 1-hour sample equals or exceeds 180 mg/dL (10 mmol/L) or the 2-hour sample equals or exceeds 153 mg/dL (8.5 mmol/L). As per the 2013 consensus of the National Institutes of Health (NIH), a two-step diagnostic criterion for GDM was developed. In this method, a 1-hour 50-gram glucose load sample is tested. If the result is greater than 140 mg/dl, a 3-hour 100-gram OGTT is recommended. The 100-gram OGTT is conducted in fasting state. The criteria were backed by the American College of Obstetricians and Gynecologists (ACOG). GDM screening should be conducted between 24–28 weeks of gestation. The two-step criteria is thought to be more beneficial than the single-step test as it does not require a fasting state, which is easier for pregnant women, and the one-step test brings more women under GDM criteria. But on the other hand, the International Association of the Diabetes and Pregnancy Study Groups (IADPSG) recommended the single step 75-gram glucose OGTT strategy to be more beneficial in terms of clinical and therapeutic outcomes. A recent study conducted in Spain demonstrated much a better result with the IADPSG criteria (one step) than the two-step criteria. The benefits were determined in terms of reduction in the rate of gestational hypertension, prematurity, caesarean section and other criteria [6, 8, 9]. For more information on diagnosis of T1DM and T2DM, readers can easily consult 'Standards of Medical Care in Diabetes – 2018' published by the American Diabetes Association; it is considered an authentic and reliable guideline.

Diabetes insipidus (DI), as described in previous chapters, is non-hyperglycaemic diabetes that is primarily characterised by excessive urine output. Diagnosis of DI is usually made with three general modalities, namely a water-deprivation test, vasopressin test and MRI scan. In the water-deprivation test, the patient is deprived of consuming water (or any liquid) for a fixed period of time and the diluted state of urine in that condition is analysed. An increased urine output is an indirect reflection of DI irrespective of the cause. The water deprivation test is considered an indirect method as any form of diuresis compromises the concentration gradient in renal medulla and in such conditions the aquaporin-2 in the kidneys get downregulated. Following that, a vasopressin test is performed in which the patient is injected with the pharmacological AVP. If excessive urine output is decreased, that means the patient is producing less endogenous AVP and is suffering from cranial or central DI. On the other hand, if the patient continues to have excessive urine output even after AVP infusion, it is an indication that the patient is producing adequate endogenous AVP, but his/her kidneys are unable to respond properly. This indicates a nephrogenic DI. Thirdly, an MRI scan is usually done to check the intensity of hypothalamic damage in the case of cranial DI [10]. Measurement of copeptin is considered to be a direct method. Copeptin is a C-terminal segment of AVP and is considered to be AVP surrogate. It has a high *ex vivo* stability that makes its assay easy. It was suggested that a copeptin level of 4.9 pmol/L or less indicated central DI, while a level more than 4.9 pmol/L is suggestive of polyuria due to primary polydipsia or nephrogenic DI [11]. Since this was reported very recently, the measurement of plasma copeptin has not achieved a clinical status as of yet.

PHARMACOLOGICAL TREATMENT OF DIABETES

The diagnosis of diabetes is followed by a treatment regimen according to the patient's condition. As per the recommendations by the ADA and also mentioned in the guidelines by the Joslin Diabetes Centre, nutritional habits and lifestyle modifications should be primarily considered before prescribing anti-hyperglycaemic medications. If the goal seems to be unmet, metformin is usually considered as the starting drug, unless and otherwise contraindicated. Starting with the treatment guidelines for T1DM patients, subcutaneous injectable insulin still remains the mainstay. The initiating dose is generally 0.4–1 unit/kg/day with a higher amount requirement during puberty. The subcutaneous insulin injection is present either as multiple daily injections or a continuous subcutaneous insulin infusion (CSII). Recently, the continuous glucose monitoring system or the hybrid closed loop system pump (MiniMed 670G by Medtronic) has been approved by the FDA. This device continuously monitors the glucose fluctuations and delivers the insulin accordingly. This control of insulin dose is done by an algorithm that is incorporated into the instrument. Details on the type of approved insulin can be found in the previous chapter on anti-diabetic drugs [6, 12]. Apart from insulin, Pramlintide is also approved for use in T1DM patients. The insulin dose needs to be adjusted when Pramlintide is recommended. Details can be found in the previous chapter on anti-diabetic drugs. Metformin, SGLT-2 inhibitors and GLP-1 analogues are being considered as adjuvant medicines but are certainly approved for use primarily in T2DM cases. Apart from these medical treatment modules, islet and pancreatic transplantation remains the current viable surgical alternative in the case of severe uncontrolled hyperglycaemia with diabetic comorbidities in T1DM patients [6]. Regarding the treatment modalities of T2DM patients, metformin is the preferred initiating therapeutic agent, if not contraindicated. Insulin is the preferred initiating agent even in newly diagnosed T2DM if the patient is symptomatic and the plasma glucose equals or exceeds the 300 mg/dL value, while the HbA1c value is greater than 10%. Metformin is considered safer than sulphonylureas as the first line of therapy considering its beneficial effect on the cardiovascular system and weight management, aside from any hypoglycaemic events. Metformin administration is rarely associated with lactic acidosis and vitamin B_{12} deficiency. Therefore, physicians must periodically keep tabs on the vitamin B_{12} level of the patient and to check of any symptoms of lactic acidosis. Dietary and lifestyle management are a must for diabetes patients and it is also recommended that strict dietary modifications and lifestyle management should be advised if the physician judiciously decides not to start the metformin (at pre-diabetes stage) [6, 13]. If the HbA1c target level (less than 7%) is not achieved after metformin monotherapy even after 3 months and the patient does not show any atherosclerotic features, a combination therapy can be initiated with a non-insulin oral anti-diabetic agent with metformin as one of the drugs. If at the initial diagnosis the HbA1c value is approximately 9%, combination therapy can be initiated with metformin being one of the agents [6, 13]. Beneficial effects of metformin can be analysed by perhaps the largest diabetes prevention trial (DPP study) which indicates that metformin reduced the incidence of diabetes by almost 31% as compared to a placebo after an average of 2.8 years of follow-up and by 18% after 15 years of the study (DPPOS analyses) [14]. Metformin is often combined with other non-insulin anti-diabetic medicine (dual therapy) if the target HbA1c goal is not achieved after 3 months of initial medical intervention. A triple oral therapy is also sometimes recommended based on the severity of the disease progression and other parameters. Insulin is often added with metformin at the initial diagnosis if the patient is symptomatic,

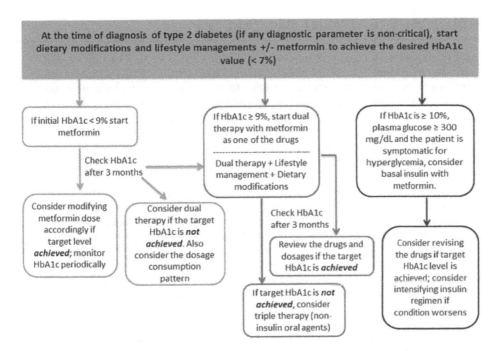

Figure 7.1 Therapeutic considerations in type 2 diabetes mellitus; referred to in References [6] and [11].

HbA1c ≥10% and FPG ≥300 mg/dL [6]. Some recently approved combination medicines include Xigduo XR (metformin + dapagliflozin), Synjardy (metformin + empagliflozin), Glyxambi (linagliptin + empagliflozin), Steglujan (ertugliflozin + sitagliptin), Segluromet (metformin + ertugliflozin) (www.healthline.com/health/diabetes/diabetes-new-drugs# new-diabetes-drugs). A brief flowchart regarding type 2 diabetes treatment modality is represented in Figure 7.1. More details about the therapeutic considerations in T1DM and T2DM are provided in the 'Standards of Medical Care in Diabetes – 2018' by the American Diabetes Association.

SURGICAL TREATMENT OF DIABETES

Aside from the pharmacological treatment, there are various surgical treatments that are preferred in extreme cases of diabetes. These surgical techniques are broadly divided into three types – pancreatic transplantation, islet transplantation and bariatric surgery. Pancreatic transplantation is done when the patient is showing repetitive episodes of hypoglycaemia with chronic other organ morbidities. It has been reported by the Diabetes Control and Complications Trial (DCCT) that T1DM patients who are on intensive insulin therapy may show considerable improvement in the rate of secondary complications of diabetes but life-threatening iatrogenic hypoglycaemia has a good chance of occurring. A pancreatic transplantation restores normal insulin signalling and action with minimal occurrence of severe hypoglycaemia with improvement of other organ function index too. Pancreatic transplantation is technically classified into three types viz. pancreatic transplantation alone (PTA), simultaneous pancreas-kidney transplantation (SPK) and pancreas after kidney transplantation (PAK). The choice is judged by the physician and performing surgeons after thorough clinical examination. The first pancreatic transplantation was performed back in 1966 by Dr William Kelly and Dr Richard Lillehei. After that, almost 80% of pancreatic transplantations have been SPK in diabetic patients with severe renal damage (uraemia); around 15% have been PAK; and only around 5% have been PTA in non-uraemic diabetic patients [15]. Bariatric surgery is often performed on morbidly obese patients with or without clinical diabetes after thorough clinical judgement by the physician and surgeons. Although, in obese subjects with symptomatic diabetes, bariatric surgery has resulted in a significant reduction in both obesity and diabetes. The surgery usually decreases the volume of the stomach and sometimes an anatomical change in the small intestine is also introduced. The major four kinds of bariatric surgeries available worldwide are gastric band, gastric bypass (Roux-en-Y gastric bypass), gastric sleeve (sleeve gastrectomy) and less commonly biliopancreatic diversion with duodenal switch. The first three lead to a decrease in the amount of food that can be consumed, while the last one usually decreases the absorption of calories and nutrients [16]. The third surgical treatment for uncontrolled diabetes with comorbidities (in both obese and non-obese subjects) is islet transplantation. In this procedure, the islets usually from a cadaver are isolated, purified, processed and finally transferred into the recipient. The islets transplantation is performed by a trained radiologist. The purified and processed islets are generally transferred into the portal veins. However, this technique is currently labelled as an 'experimental procedure' by the FDA until sufficient evidence of a greater benefit-to-risk ratio is obtained in order to term it a 'treatment'. As it is currently under experimental protocol, only autograft and allograft are permitted [17].

Pancreatic transplantation alone or PTA is, according to a few reports, presently the least opted-for procedure because there is a very high chance that the patient may require a renal transplant in the near future due to grafting technicalities and use of immunosuppressive drugs. PTA is, however, the preferred choice for patients who are unaware of their hypoglycaemic state, but have a stable renal condition and minimum proteinuria. It was reported that nearly 30% of PTA patients would need a renal transplant due to serious nephrotoxicity by the immunosuppressive drug class of calcineurin inhibitors (CIs; cyclosporine and tacrolimus), which are very commonly used to prevent the graft rejection. But this severe toxicity of CIs is very difficult to avoid currently. But PTA still remains the procedure of choice for T1DM patients with brittle diabetes but very early or no renal dysfunction [18]. With conflicting PTA outcomes in different reports, a recent meta-analysis emphasised that PTA is still a beneficial and successful procedure in terms of comparative outcomes. It stated that the risk of death following PTA is less than 2%, which is even less than the percentage of subjects waiting for a pancreatic transplant. As part of an interesting analysis, it stated that the overall mortality globally for T1DM patients is 812 patients per 100,000 per year, while the figure is just 320 per 100,000 patients per year for the patients receiving PTA. Indicating the problem of nephrotoxicity, it stated that currently more PTA patients receive a comparatively safer combination of tacrolimus and mycophenolate mofetil immunosuppressive drugs. Further, regarding the rate of renal transplant following a PTA, it was reported that in the period between 1994–1997, 21% of patients received a renal transplant within 5 years of PTA that significantly improved to 6% between the period 2002–2007. It was also reported that in the period between 2002 and 2011, the need for further renal transplantation in PTA patients decreased to 6% 5 years after PTA [15]. The use of calcineurin inhibitors and the resultant development of renal toxicity leading to renal damage were further confirmed in a very recent patient study by Shin et al. [19]. They emphasised in their trial that the use of tacrolimus, a calcineurin inhibitor, was the only significant factor that caused the end-stage renal disease (ERSD). As a general observation, a report published in The Lancet almost a decade ago reported that patients with an eGFR between 80–100 mL/min/1.73 m^2 undergoing PTA were unlikely to require a renal transplant in the future. Those who had an eGFR less than 80 mL/min/1.73 m^2 undergoing PTA might need a renal transplant 10 years after the procedure. However, patients with an eGFR of less than 50–60 mL/min/1.73 m^2 have a very high chance of a renal transplant before PTA, during PTA or just after PTA [20].

In a recent report by Fridell et al. [21], it is reported that for T1DM patients with uraemia, PAK should be the preferred pancreatic transplant procedure. As per the report, it is stated that on grafting terms, PTA is better than SPK because it is widely accepted that a living donor renal transplantation has a better allograft result and patient compliance as compared to a cadaveric donor. This is because in SPK, both the pancreas and kidney are usually from cadaveric donors. It was reported, however, that the risk of pancreatic graft rejection was similar in both PAK and SPK. In PAK, the baseline immunosuppressive drugs that are already in action might help in the better acceptance of a pancreas. However, as patients awaiting PAK are already immunosuppressed, they have a very high chance of acquiring a post-surgical infection. Secondly, a second surgical procedure is definitely not patient compliant for those awaiting PAK. A few centres, however, completely eliminated the need for a second surgery by performing simultaneous cadaveric pancreas transplantation living donor kidney grafting (SPLK) and have achieved excellent results. Although the rate of graft rejection has seen a significant decrease in the case of PAK in the last 20 years, it is almost the same for SPK. However, the administration of newer immunosuppressive drugs (anti-thymocyte antibodies and mycophenolate mofetil) without any calcineurin inhibitors has made the grafts safer and longer lasting.

Regarding SPK, as per our current review of available literature, it is the most common procedure applied to brittle diabetic patients with severe renal dysfunction awaiting a pancreatic transplantation. On a technical front, different transplantation centres may have different surgical procedures, but most of them utilise the intraperitoneal segment for graft placement. While the pancreas is grafted into the right iliac fossa, the renal grafting is performed at contralateral iliac fossa. This procedure is said to be associated with less fluid accumulation around the grafted pancreas and better post-surgical wound healing [22]. Even in terms of using thymoglobulin (anti-human thymocyte antibody for T-cell depletion) for renal transplantation, it was reported that PTA patients received the highest dose, while SPK patients received the lowest dose [20]. But a few recent analyses have reported that PAK has a much better survival rate compared to T1DM patients with uraemia who are waiting for SPK [23–25]. Therefore, it can be interpreted based on various post-surgical meta-analyses that for patients who are awaiting a SPK with a waiting time more than 1 year, a PAK would be a better and feasible alternative if a living renal donor is available.

Islet transplantation is comparatively new to the pancreatic transplantation procedures. The first reported islet transplantation, known as the Edmonton Protocol, was performed by Shapiro et al. in 2000 in Canada. They used a combination of sirolimus, low-dose tacrolimus and an IL-2 receptor monoclonal antibody (daclizumab) for immunosuppression. They removed the glucocorticoids as one of the immunosuppressives owing to its hyperglycaemic effects. The choice of graft site was the portal veins. There were no islet rejections while the median hospital stay was 2.3 days, which is much less than that required for pancreatic transplantations. Sirolimus was used as it has a much less reported nephrotoxicity as compared to tacrolimus [26]. The islet transplantation is again the treatment of choice as it is minimally invasive in nature and is associated with much less morbidity as compared to whole pancreatic transplantation. Generally, two or three islet infusions (each infusion generally contains around 5,000 cells/kg body weight) are enough to meet the required metabolic and therapeutic criteria. Most patients require exogenous insulin after 5 years of the transplantation procedure as the graft function starts to decline. Even with surgical and therapeutic benefits, islet transplantation has not become a treatment of choice for uncontrolled and comorbid T1DM because of scarcity of living donors, high cost of cell isolation and maintenance of high-skilled laboratory for such a procedure. The procedure is, therefore, reserved for almost the same set of patients as in case of pancreatic transplantation. As this is not yet an approved 'therapy', patients undergoing such procedures are mostly assigned to a clinical trial after proper informed consent. In the UK in particular, islet transplantation is becoming a treatment of choice for those who already had a kidney transplant and are on immunosuppressive drugs. In a trial reported by the multi-centric Collaborative Islet Transplant Registry (CITR) for 257 islet transplant recipients between 1999 and 2008, after 3 years, almost 27% patients were confirmed insulin independent, while C-peptide was detected in almost 57% of the patients. It is also reported that islet transplantation improved diabetes-related micro- and macro-vascular complications, such as nephropathy and retinopathy. The most opted site of islet transplantation is the portal vein from where the islets reach the liver. But the major problems faced by islets at the liver site are high concentration of glucose and immunoreaction. Though immunosuppressives are administered, certain immunosuppressives such as calcineurin inhibitors and steroids damage the islets. Secondly, after purification and processing, the final number of islets (though transfused around 5,000 cells/kg body weight) does not bring the required improvement and, thus, two or three infusions are required. Though islet transplantation is done laparoscopically, one of the major surgical complications that might occur if proper precautions and steps are not taken, is the hepatic bleeding that occurs during the catheterisation of the trans-hepatic portal vein; however, with proper use of gelatine plugs (Gelfoam) and fibrin sealants, this has now been significantly minimised [27]. Islet transplantation, particularly in the case of autografting, is particularly beneficial on the immunological front because the patient will receive his/her own pancreatic cells after purification and selection. In such a case, there is no need for the use of immunosuppressive drugs. On the other hand, it has been reported that many immunosuppressive drugs that are used for islet allograft are themselves toxic to the insulin-producing β-cells. This situation arose mostly because of the use of steroid and calcineurin inhibitors after islet grafting. But with the use of newer and comparatively safer immunosuppressives, toxicity towards β-cells has been minimised. In islet transplantation, glucagon-producing α-cells are also grafted. It has been reported that since the intrahepatic site is the most common site for such a procedure and there is a constant glycogenesis and glucose flux, transplanted α-cells fail to recognise the blood sugar level and do not respond accordingly, failing to release glucagon. But when the islets were experimentally grafted to non-hepatic sites, the glucagon secretion and response were close to normal. It was also observed in such experiments that there is a partial glucagon release when the blood glucose level goes below 50 mg/dL. This mild glucagon release response was shown to occur due to the action of epinephrine. Thus, it would be logically, and to some extent scientifically, good to transplant an equal amount of islets at the non-hepatic site too [28]. The importance of islet autotransplantation can be analysed by a recent report that examines the possible therapeutic outcome in 409 T1DM patients who received a total pancreatectomy with islet autotransplantation (TPIAT). It stated that with the use of almost 5,000 islets/kg body weight (approximately 350,000 islets or one-third of the physiological number), almost 93% of patients achieved and maintained their HbA1c <7% at the third-year follow-up with a 71% level of insulin independence. One of the reasons stated is the 'freshness' of the islets because the place of surgical removal of the pancreas and the place of islet isolation and processing were in the same location. Thus, the conditions of islets from a cadaver, the time of their transport to the islet-processing laboratory and again the time for islets to reach the final destination were greatly bypassed. Secondly, islet autotransplantation eliminates the need for immunosuppressive drugs and this becomes a boon for the patients. Thus, autotransplantation of islets can prove to be much more beneficial as compared to islet allotransplantation when the pancreatectomy could be a logical choice in brittle T1DM patients, provided that non-hepatic sites are also considered for autotransplantation to restore the normal functioning and sensing of α-cells to sense hypoglycaemia correctly [29]. In another promising study, perhaps the first randomised multi-centric study for islet allotransplantation (TRIMECO trial), it was shown that there was a very significant metabolic improvement in patients with islet transplantation as compared to those who were on insulin regimen. Almost 93% patients who received islets had a functional graft after 12 months with a median HbA1c <5.8%. The severe and frequent hypoglycaemic episodes before transplantation improved significantly after the procedure as compared to the group that was on insulin therapy. A total of 11,000 islets/kg body weight was infused in two to three infusions. Almost 59% of transplant group patients were insulin independent after 12 months. All these patients who received an islet allotransplant had a kidney transplant prior to the islet graft, and it was seen that the renal function improved significantly after the islet transplantation. But the major adverse events that were recorded were bleeding (7% of patients at 6 months and 6% of patients at 12 months), haemorrhage (6% of patients at 12 months) and portal thrombosis (in one patient). A large percentage did show a high HLA antibody generation that is not a good indication in case they need a future islet transplant. Though based on a very small patient number (total recorded 46 patients), the TRIMECO trial shows a high degree of positivity for islet transplantation in patients who have brittle diabetes and previously had a renal transplant [30].

Now coming to bariatric surgery, as stated above, it is basically a surgery carried out to treat morbid obesity, but its metabolic effects on T2DM have been significant. Gastric bypass, also known as Roux-en-Y gastric bypass (RYGB), is often considered as the gold standard among all the obesity corrective surgical measures. This method, briefly, is done in two parts. In the first part, the stomach is stapled so that two pouches of different sizes are formed. In the second part, the small intestine is cut and its lower end (jejunum) is sutured to the small segment of the stomach. This procedure has two major effects – the amount of food that can be consumed becomes lower due to the size of the modified stomach, and secondly due to less stay time in the small intestine, fewer calories are absorbed. The rerouting not only affects the food volume but also modifies the gut hormone and probiotic bacteria so that satiety is controlled. This procedure could possibly reduce almost 50% of the body weight, but the long hospital stay, and vitamin/mineral deficiency are the major drawbacks. The RYGB method reduces hyperglycaemia due to lower food and calorie intake. In a second method called sleeve gastrectomy or simply sleeve, almost 80% of the stomach is removed, while the remaining part looks like a banana in shape. This method also aims at reducing the volume of food intake. This is a completely irreversible surgery. Because of lowered caloric intake, this method is also highly useful in controlling diabetes. In a third method called gastric banding, an inflatable band is tied across the stomach so that a small and a large pouch are created. This again leads to lowering the food volume and produces early satiety. The size of the channel opening between the small and large gastric pouch can be controlled by inflating it with normal saline. There is comparatively much less malabsorption of the nutrients and the process is reversible as compared to the other two methods. A fourth surgical procedure, known as duodenal switch, is usually not preferred for various surgical reasons [31, 32]. In a meta-analysis more than a decade ago, it was reported that out of the data analysed for 1,846 patients, 1,417 patients (76.8%) displayed complete amelioration of diabetes (T2DM). This effect on diabetes was observed as a result of loss of central obesity and changes in the gut hormone secretion and action. In the analysis, the diabetes reversal was found in 83.7% patients who had a gastric bypass, in around 71% who underwent a gastrectomy and in around 48% patients in the gastric banding group. There was also a drastic improvement in the lipid profile of the patients, while almost 61.7% of the patients displayed significant improvement in hypertension [33]. A similar significant T2DM control after RYGB was shown in a recent meta-analysis too [34]. Apart from the reduction in food volume and calorie absorption, another special metabolic effect observed especially with gastric bypass or RYGB is the exceedingly high surge of GLP-1. Since we know GLP-1 is a strong insulinotropic hormone, the reduction in hyperglycaemia is not only due to calorie restriction, but also, significantly, due to the metabolic action of GLP-1. Secondly, metabolic calorie restriction is also observed as an important effect of GLP-1. The basis of this observation was that the researchers at different centres observed that severe hypoglycaemia was present in many patients who underwent RYGB and their plasma GLP-1 level was almost 10–20 times higher than normal [35]. The RYGB procedure not only has an effect on GLP-1 but also on other gastric hormones. RYGB has been reported to have structural and anatomical changes in gut lining too by possible induction of chronic and atrophic gastritis with a marked reduction in the G-cells. G-cells are responsible for the secretion of the gut hormone gastrin. Therefore, it is seen that RYGB led to a significant decrease in post-prandial gastrin production and secretion coupled with excess acid production in the stomach which result in the alteration of histological features. On the other hand, there are few reports that sleeve gastrectomy increases gastrin level, the reason for which is not clear. Ghrelin is an orexigenic hormone (stimulating hunger) that is secreted from the stomach and pancreas in response to hunger and decreases upon eating. Fasting and caloric restriction are said to increase the ghrelin level. But in a study involving subjects who underwent gastric banding and RYGB compared to control subjects who were under dietary management, it was seen that where gastric banding and dietary restrictions increase the ghrelin level, RYGB was associated with decreased ghrelin production. Though theoretically contradictory, this effect was concluded due to an absence of direct contact between the ghrelin-producing area and the food nutrients. A similar effect of decreased ghrelin was also observed after a sleeve gastrectomy. The hormone cholecystokinin (CCK) is released from I-cells in the duodenum as a stimulus to the dietary constituents or due to parasympathetic regulation. The exact reason for increased CCK after RYGB is still not very clear; however, a possible mechanism suggests a physiological change in CCK-producing cells post RYGB. The effect of high CCK post RYGB and sleeve gastrectomy is seen as increased satiety and improved blood glucose regulation. Post-prandial release of glucose-dependent insulinotropic polypeptide (GIP; secreted from K-cells) from the duodenum and jejunum results in insulin secretion to regulate the blood glucose. Bariatric surgical processes such as RYGB and sleeve gastrectomy significantly reduce the GIP production and thus post-prandial insulin regulation may be hampered. Despite a loss in GIP production and secretion, there is a considerable improvement in T2DM post-bariatric surgeries that is possibly due to more prominent effect of high GLP-1. The reason for this increased GLP-1 is not very clear, but could be attributed to direct contact of intact nutrients with the ileum due to the surgical rerouting. It was also noticed that the blood level of GLP-1 was high in patients who responded well and lost large amounts of weight after RYGB as compared to those who did not lose much weight [36, 37]. Peptide YY (PYY) is another hormone released by L-cells that, after being cleaved by DPP-4, get converted to its active form and promotes satiety through its agonist action on Y2 receptors. Though it has a role in delaying gastric emptying, its primary action is thought to be the central action of appetite. It has also been observed that obese people have less PYY, while it is present in a higher amount in lean people. RYGB, gastric banding and sleeve gastrectomy all resulted in a significant increase in PYY even after a year of surgery. Thus, this is also one of the possible mechanisms of the beneficial effects of bariatric surgery [36, 37]. Oxyntomodulin is another hormonal peptide released post-prandially from L-cells that has a significant weight loss effect owing to promotion of satiety. It has been observed that obese T2DM patients who underwent RYGB had a significant increase in their oxyntomodulin level as compared to matched patients who had diet-restricted weight reduction. But the exact mechanism of how bariatric surgeries influence the release of oxyntomodulin is still a matter of research. In obese patients with T2DM, insulin resistance is very common. It has been shown that after bariatric procedures, the serum insulin level decreases significantly to near normal levels, while there is a positive modulation of insulin sensitivity The effect of RYGB and sleeve gastrectomy was also quite significantly positive towards the overall β-cell functions [36, 37]. The metabolic improvement results of bariatric surgery are not only based upon positive alteration of gut hormone but owe a lot to the shift in the colonisation of different species of gut microbiota. In an interesting study recently published, it was observed that the pre-surgery obese subjects had major colonisation of Clostridial clusters consisting of species such as *Roseburia* and *Ruminococcus* that can ferment carbohydrates to butyrate and acetate, while the gut microbiota in post-bariatric surgery patients shifted to species such as *Lactobacillus*, *Megasphaera elsdenii* and *Streptococcus*. This shift of microbial population from obese to post-surgical patients suggested a more important role of production of short-chain fatty acids that is quite helpful in gut hormone secretion [38]. Aside from this finding, Zhang et al. [39] showed almost a decade ago that obese individuals display a high colonisation of hydrogen-producing bacteria of the Prevotellaceae (a subgroup of Bacteroidetes) and Fermicutes family and co-existence of the hydrogen-oxidising methanogenic *Archaea* species. While it was observed that the normal weight and post-surgery subjects had no methanogens in the intestine with a significant decrease in the population of Fermicutes. Thus, not limited to the results discussed, we can find that physiological and metabolic improvements after bariatric surgeries owe a lot to the positive change in the gut hormones and the microbiota colonising the gut.

Aside from these conventional surgical measures to treat diabetes and obesity, research is in full swing for transplantation of encapsulated islets. Microencapsulation of cells is a technique whereby the cells of interest are encapsulated inside a semi-permeable membrane of a biopolymer that protects the cell from graft rejection but permits the movement of nutrients inside, while that of the therapeutic product outside. As with all other transplants, islet transplant is also associated with graft rejection and use of immunosuppressants. To overcome this scenario, researchers have developed techniques to encapsulate islets inside biopolymer microspheres such that the cells remain viable and do not encounter immune rejection. The opening of this gateway is mostly credited to a work by Lim et al. in 1980 [40]. They encapsulated the β-cells in alginate microspheres and were able to show their functionality intact for 4 months. Among all the research about islet encapsulation, probably the first report of clinical use was published in 2007. In this 10-year-long study, a T1DM patient was implanted with alginate-encapsulated porcine islets (15,000 islets/kg body weight) intraperitoneally. Although the experiment wasn't entirely scientifically successful, it opened up the path for more clinical study with encapsulated allo- and xenotransplantation [41]. ViaCyte, a California-based regenerative medicine company, has devised a polymeric retrievable device named Encaptra with stems cells that have been differentiated into precursor islet cells (named PEC-Encap or VC-01). The device is implanted subcutaneously as this site is considered to be better than the peritoneal site (due to gravitation effect at intraperitoneal space). In a 2-year phase 1/2 clinical trial on 19 patients very recently reported (STEP ONE trial), it was shown that the device was completely safe, and the therapeutic delivery was well maintained. The device also allowed a significant vasculature around it, which is a good sign. The researchers also noted the absence of any autoantibodies or alloantibodies in the patients' circulation. This is the first human trial with a stem-cell-derived pancreatic islet transplant [42]. Aside from all of this 'biological' research about transplanting encapsulated islets, Medtronic, one of the world's largest medical device companies based in Dublin, Ireland, has devised a hybrid closed-loop insulin delivery system known as the MINIMED 670G SYSTEM. A hybrid closed-loop system is one that senses the biomarker (in this case, blood glucose) and delivers the therapeutic product (in this case, insulin) as per the need. The MINIMED 670G is the world's first such system to receive FDA approval [43]. The MINIMED 670G operates on a novel 'SmartGuard Technology' that senses the glucose fluctuation every 5–10 minutes and adjusts the basal insulin delivery as per the reading. This glucose reading is based on a continuous glucose monitoring (CGM) system. This kind of bolus insulin adjustment mimics the pancreatic function to the nearest physiological state possible. Such a system is very useful in preventing the hypoglycaemic episodes that can be dangerous at times if hypoglycaemia unawareness is present. The device stops delivering insulin when the glucose level is detected below the lower limit and automatically starts controlled insulin delivery once it detects that the glucose level is high enough for insulin [44, 45]. Apart from Medtronic's device, there are a few other CGM and hybrid closed-loop (HCL) devices. These are the Free Style Libre System (CGM; Abbott), G4 Platinum (CGM; Dexcom), G5 Mobile (CGM; Dexcom), MiniMed 530G, 630G, Paradigm Revel (HCL; Medtronic), T-slim X2 (HCL; TandemDiabetes Care) and One Touch Vibe™ Plus (HCL with G5 Dexcom; Johnson & Johnson). The G5 system from Dexcom is a mobile application based CGM system and the T-slim X2 HCL is an insulin pump connected to the G5 CGM system [46, 47]. In addition to these CGM and HCL systems, a company called PKvitality uses a microneedle-based 'wristwatch'-like wearable biosensor that measures glucose from the interstitial fluid. The product is marketed as the K'Watch Glucose and is again a CGM system [48]. Regarding the basic science of CGM systems, a tiny sensor is usually placed under the abdominal skin or the skin of arm. This sensor continuously measures the glucose level from the interstitial fluid. The transmitter, collecting the information from the sensor, transmits the information to the associated monitor. This monitor might be associated to the insulin pump (in an HCL system) or works just as a 'monitor' (in a CGM system) and could even be a part of a mobile device (as in the G5 Dexcom system) [49].

Thus, both biological systems and electronic devices have shown promise in the treatment of diabetes. If pharmacological treatments become unresponsive and the patient reaches a state of periodic hypoglycaemia with hypoglycaemia unawareness, pancreatic or islet transplantation is often suggested. Although there have been good results with these transplants, the use of immunosuppressives become a significant problem for patients as well as the gradual graft failure (if any). To avoid the use of immunosuppressive drugs and promote the xenograft (since live and cadaveric donors are scarce), islet microencapsulation has been tested as the treatment of choice. Microencapsulation significantly reduces the immune rejection of the transplanted islets and removes the use of lifelong immunosuppressive drugs. Research is still ongoing with the encapsulating material and site of transplant, and on the commercial front, ViaCyte has delivered a ray of hope with its PEC-Encap system, which has recently completed a phase 1/2 trial with positive reports. Research is never ending, and more research is certainly needed to counter a global epidemic of a multifactorial disease such as diabetes.

REFERENCES

1. Accessed at www.who.int/diabetes/action_online/basics/en/index1.html; accessed on August 19, 2018.
2. Ramachandran A. Know the signs and symptoms of diabetes. *Indian J Med Res* 2014;140(5):579–581.
3. Accessed at www.hopkinsguides.com/hopkins/view/Johns_Hopkins_Diabetes_Gu ide/547013/all/Autoantibodies_in_Type_1_Diabetes#18176860; accessed on August 19, 2018.
4. Wenzlau JM, Hutton JC. Novel diabetes autoantibodies and prediction of type 1 diabetes. *Curr Diab Rep* 2013;13(5):608–615.
5. Calderon B, Sacks DB. Islet autoantibodies and type 1 diabetes: Does the evidence support screening? *Clin Chem* 2014;60(3):438–440.
6. American Diabetes Association. Classification and diagnosis of diabetes: Standards of medical care in diabetes-2018. *Diabetes Care* 2018;41(Suppl 1):S13–S27.
7. Accessed at www.joslin.org/docs/CLINICAL-GUIDELINE-FOR-ADULTS-WITH-DIABE TES-Rev-05-17-2017.pdf; accessed on August 19, 2018.
8. Khalafallah A, Phuah E, Al-Barazan AM, Nikakis I, Radford A, Clarkson W et al. Glycosylated haemoglobin for screening and diagnosis of gestational diabetes mellitus. *BMJ Open* 2016;6(4):e011059.
9. Duran A, Saenz S, Torrejon MJ, Bordeu E, del Valle L, Galindo M et al. Introduction of IADPSG criteria for the screening and diagnosis of gestational diabetes mellitus results in improved pregnancy outcomes at a lower cost in a large cohort of pregnant women: The St. Carlos gestational diabetes study. *Diabetes Care* 2014;37(9):2442–2450.

10. Accessed at www.nhs.uk/conditions/diabetes-insipidus/diagnosis/.
11. Fenske W, Refardt J, Chifu I, Schnyder I, Winzeler B, Drummond J et al. A copeptin-based approach in the diagnosis of diabetes insipidus. *N Engl J Med* 2018;379(5):428–439.
12. Accessed at www.ncbi.nlm.nih.gov/books/NBK476442/.
13. Canadian Diabetes Association. Pharmacologic management of type 2 diabetes: 2016 Interim update. *Can J Diabetes* 2016;40(3):193–195.
14. Aroda VR, Knowler WC, Crandall JP, Perreault L, Edelstein SL, Jeffries SL et al. Metformin for diabetes prevention: Insights gained from the Diabetes Prevention Program/Diabetes Prevention Program Outcomes Study. *Diabetologia* 2017;60(9):1601–1611.
15. Gruessner RWG, Gruessner AC. Pancreas transplant alone: A procedure coming of age. *Diabetes Care* 2013;36(8):2440–2447.
16. Accessed at www.niddk.nih.gov/health-information/weight-management/bariatric-surgery/types; accessed on October 6, 2018.
17. Accessed at www.niddk.nih.gov/health-information/diabetes/overview/insulin-medicines-treatments/pancreatic-islet-transplantation; accessed on October 6, 2018.
18. Hampson FA, Freeman SJ, Ertner J, Drage M, Butler A, Watson CJ et al. Pancreatic transplantation: Surgical technique, normal radiological appearances and complications. *Insights Imaging* 2010;1(5–6):339–347.
19. Shin S, Jung CH, Choi JY, Kwon HW, Jung JH, Kim YH et al. Long-term effects of pancreas transplant alone on nephropathy in type 1 diabetic patients with optimal renal function. *PLoS One* 2018;13(1):e0191421.
20. White SA, Shaw JA, Sutherland DER. Pancreas transplantation. *Lancet* 2009;373(9677):1808–1817.
21. Fridell JA, Powelson JA. Pancreas after kidney transplantation: Why is the most logical option the least popular? *Curr Opin Organ Transplant* 2015;20(1):108 – 114.
22. Jiang AT, Rowe N, Sener A, Luke P. Simultaneous pancreas-kidney transplantation: The role in the treatment of type 1 diabetes and end-stage renal disease. *Can Urol Assoc J* 2014;8(3-4):135–138.
23. Fridell JA, Niederhaus S, Curry M, Urban R, Fox A, Odorico J. The survival advantage of pancreas after kidney transplant. *Am J Transplant* 2018. doi:10.1111/ajt.15106. [Epub ahead of print].
24. Accessed at https://optn.transplant.hrsa.gov/media/2348/pancreas_guidance_201712.pdf; accessed on October 6, 2018.
25. Ito T, Kenmochi T, Aida N, Kurihara K, Kawai A, Ito T. A study of effectiveness of preceding solo-kidney transplantation for type 1 diabetes with end stage renal failure. *Transplant Proceed* 2018. doi:10.1016/j.transproceed.2018.06.014.
26. Shapiro AM, Lakey JR, Ryan EA, Korbutt GS, Toth E, Warnock GL et al. Islet transplantation in seven patients with type 1 diabetes mellitus using a glucocorticoid-free immunosuppressive regimen. *N Engl J Med* 2000;343(4):230–238.
27. de Kort H, de Koning EJ, Rabelink TJ, Bruijn JA, Bajema IM. Islet transplantation in type 1 diabetes. *BMJ* 2011;342:d217.
28. Robertson RP. Islet transplantation for type 1 diabetes, 2015: What have we learned from alloislet and autoislet successes? *Diabetes Care* 2015;38(6):1030–1035.
29. Robertson RP. Spontaneous hypoglycemia after islet transplantation: The case for using non-hepatic sites. *J Clin Endocrinol Metab* 2016;101(10):3571–3574.

30. Lablanche S, Vantyghem MC, Kessler L, Wojtusciszyn A, Borot S, Thivolet C et al. Islet transplantation versus insulin therapy in patients with type 1 diabetes with severe hypoglycaemia or poorly controlled glycaemia after kidney transplantation (TRIMECO): A multicentre, randomised controlled trial. *Lancet Diabetes Endocrinol* 2018;6(7):527–537.
31. Accessed at https://asmbs.org/patients/bariatric-surgery-procedures.
32. Accessed at www.niddk.nih.gov/health-information/weight-management/bariatric-surgery/types.
33. Buchwald H, Avidor Y, Braunwald E, Jensen MD, Pories W, Fahrbach K et al. Bariatric surgery: A systematic review and meta-analysis. *JAMA* 2004;292(14):1724–1737.
34. Beaulac J, Sandre D. Critical review of bariatric surgery, medically supervised diets, and behavioural interventions for weight management in adults. *Perspect Public Health* 2017;137(3):162–172.
35. Holst JJ, Madsbad S. Mechanisms of surgical control of type 2 diabetes: GLP-1 is key factor. *Surg Obes Relat Dis* 2016;12(6):1236–1242.
36. Meek CL, Lewis HB, Reimann F, Gribble FM, Park AJ. The effect of bariatric surgery on gastrointestinal and pancreatic peptide hormones. *Peptides* 2016;77:28–37.
37. Dimitriadis GK, Randeva MS, Miras AD. Potential hormone mechanisms of bariatric surgery. *Curr Obes Rep* 2017;6(3):253–265.
38. Federico A, Dallio M, Tolone S, Gravina AG, Patrone V, Romano M et al. Gastrointestinal hormones, intestinal microbiota and metabolic homeostasis in obese patients: Effect of bariatric surgery. *In Vivo* 2016;30(3):321–330.
39. Zhang H, DiBaise JK, Zuccolo A, Kudrna D, Braidotti M, Yu Y et al. Human gut microbiota in obesity and after gastric bypass. *Proc Natl Acad Sci U S A* 2009;106(7):2365–2370.
40. Lim F, Sun A. Microencapsulated islets as bioartificial endocrine pancreas. *Science* 1980;210(4472):908–910.
41. Elliott RB, Escobar L, Tan PLJ, Muzina M, Zwain S, Buchanan C. Live encapsulated porcine islets from a type 1 diabetic patient 9.5 yr after xenotransplantation. *Xenotransplantation* 2007;14(2):157–161.
42. Pullen LC. Stem cell-derived pancreatic progenitor cells have now been transplanted into patients: Report from IPITA 2018. *Am J Transplant* 2018;18(7):1581–1582.
43. Accessed at www.medtronicdiabetes.com/blog/fda-approves-minimed-670g-system-worlds-first-hybrid-closed-loop-system/.
44. Accessed at https://professional.medtronicdiabetes.com/minimed-670g-insulin-pump-system.
45. Accessed at www.fda.gov/MedicalDevices/ProductsandMedicalProcedures/DeviceApprovalsandClearances/Recently-ApprovedDevices/ucm600603.htm.
46. Accessed at http://main.diabetes.org/dforg/pdfs/2018/2018-cg-continuous-glucose-monitors.pdf.
47. Accessed at www.jnj.com/media-center/press-releases/onetouch-vibe-plus-insulin-pump-earns-fda-approval-and-health-canada-license-and-is-first-pump-integrated-with-the-dexcom-g5-mobile-continuous-glucose-monitor.
48. Accessed at www.pkvitality.com/ktrack-glucose/.
49. Accessed at www.niddk.nih.gov/health-information/diabetes/overview/managing-diabetes/continuous-glucose-monitoring.

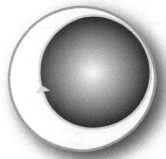

8 Dietary and Lifestyle Management of Diabetes

IMPORTANCE OF DIETARY AND LIFESTYLE MANAGEMENT IN DIABETES

As we have seen in the previous chapter, it is widely accepted and recommended that dietary modifications and lifestyle management are essential in managing the damaging effects of diabetes. Patients are almost always given the same advice along with the required medications. Since the pattern of diabetes is primarily linked to carbohydrate and fat intake, diet and lifestyle management can prove to be a boon for patients with diabetes. Perhaps the first large-scale clinical trial for validating the hypothesis that dietary and lifestyle management could reverse the diabetic condition was initiated in 1996 and finally reported in 2002 under the name of the Diabetes Prevention Program (DPP). The report was highly encouraging with the view that the T2DM incidence was reduced by almost 58% with lifestyle interventions as opposed to 31% by metformin. These results were similar across all ethnic groups and races in both male and female participants. It was also reported through the DPP study that the average fasting plasma glucose value came out to be similar with both lifestyle interventions and metformin therapy, while the HbA1c value was significantly much lower in the lifestyle intervention group than the metformin group. This suggests that dietary and lifestyle modifications can have a more pronounced positive effect in controlling plasma glucose for a longer period of time [1, 2]. It was also reported in the DPP study that while metformin can delay the progression of diabetes by 7.9%, lifestyle management can do that by an excellent figure of 20.2% [3]. In another recent study to verify the DPP program, known as the DPP Outcomes Study or DPPOS, it was reported that lifestyle intervention and metformin could delay the progression of diabetes for almost 15 years, but many participants developed diabetes after that. Moreover, lifestyle modifications and metformin were able to significantly reduce the diabetes-related microvascular complications [4]. As stated in previous chapters, diabetes has a strong positive relation to inflammation. Inflammatory markers such as C-reactive protein (CRP), IL-6 and TNF-α have been found to be elevated in patients with diabetes and have a cause–effect relationship with diabetes. It has been demonstrated that a low-fat, low-carbohydrate and high-protein diet significantly reduces the inflammatory markers in humans. A diet high in mono-unsaturated fatty acids (MUFA) and poly-unsaturated fatty acids (PUFA) results in decreased inflammation and inflammatory markers. It was also reported that the Mediterranean diet has a profound effect in decreasing inflammatory markers and HbA1c significantly in the diabetic population. In general, the Mediterranean diet is composed of six servings of vegetables and three servings of fruit per day along with fish served five to six times per week. Another important diet plan was the DASH diet or Dietary Approaches to Stop Hypertension, which comprises high intake of whole grains, vegetables and fruit and very limited salt intake [5]. As per the recent ADA report, higher consumption of nuts, yoghurt, berries, tea and coffee can reduce the risk and progression of diabetes, while red meat and sweetened sugary beverages and foods do the reverse. On the physical activity front, the ADA also suggests at least 150 minutes per week of exercise, as brisk walking can improve insulin sensitivity and decrease the progression of diabetes. Resistance training is advised to be beneficial for pre-diabetic and moderately diabetic people, while prolonged sitting or a sedentary position should be avoided [1]. The vast majority of patients with type 2 diabetes initially had pre-diabetes. Their blood glucose levels where higher than normal, but not high enough to merit a diabetes diagnosis. The cells in the body were becoming resistant to insulin. Studies have indicated that even at the pre-diabetes stage, some damage to the circulatory system and the heart may have already occurred.

In a study conducted a decade ago, it was reported that diets high in wholegrain foods and very low in processed foods and soft drinks had significant positive effect on insulin resistance, T2DM and overall metabolic syndrome. As a special consideration, it was shown that consumption of normal and diet soft drinks had a positive correlation with the incidence of diabetes [6]. According to a recent report, it has been very difficult, however, to come to a convergent point regarding the dietary recommendations for pre-diabetic and diabetic populations. For macronutrient proportions, the European and Canadian diets promotes 45–60% of energy from carbohydrate sources, 10–20% of protein and less than 35% of fat content per day, while the Indian dietary recommendations suggest 50–60% of daily energy from carbohydrate sources, 10–15% protein and fat consumption to be less than 30% per day. But the ADA suggests that there is no one recommended dietary plan. There have been reports that a low-carbohydrate food is much better than a low-fat food for weight control, while others also stress the quality of fat in a sense that MUFA and PUFA are much better than saturated fats for the diabetes population. It was also reported that low-calorie diets significantly reduced fasting plasma glucose in the diabetes population even after discontinuation of metformin. Also, a gap in calorie intake had a significant effect on the fat content of the liver and pancreas which resulted in significant glucose regulation and glucose-stimulated insulin release. It was also reported that a low-calorie dietary pattern not only controlled glucose levels but long-term glucose regulation following such a dietary plan resulted in significant reduction of diabetic complications too [7]. An overweight or obese condition is often treated as one of the most impelling factors for the development of diabetes and they have a positive correlation. As a general concept, the positive correlation between body mass index (BMI) and diabetes is greater in women than in men. It was noted from the Nurses' Health Study (NHS) that the risk ratio for diabetes development was 38.8 for people with a BMI >35, while it was 20.1 for people with a BMI between 30 and 35 as compared to people with a normal BMI. It was also observed that women who were able to lose more than 5 kg of weight within 10 years reduced the incidence and development of diabetes by 50% or more. A great positive association has also been observed between physical exercise and the risk of diabetes development. Although there are conflicting results relating to the consumption of total carbohydrates and the incidence of diabetes, the quality of carbohydrate does affect the incidence and development of diabetes. The four cardinal parameters related to the carbohydrate quality are the fibre quality and quantity, wholegrain seeds, glycaemic index (GI) and consumption of simple refined sugar items. Dietary fibre makes up the indigestible part of total carbohydrate consumption and it has been shown in various observational studies that high-fibre content in the daily diet can significantly reduce the development of obesity and diabetes. Wholegrain fibres that are slowly digested reduce the time of glucose entry into the systemic circulation and wholegrain items have also been shown to have a positive effect on gut probiotics and a negative effect on the pro-inflammatory markers. Glycaemic index or the GI shows the effect of the food item in raising the blood sugar directly when compared to a standard (generally white bread). Thus, a high-GI food will raise the blood sugar more rapidly as compared to a low-GI item. It has also been seen that the quality of fat is very effective in controlling obesity and related diabetes. Plant fat and proteins have been treated as much safer than their animal counterparts. In most randomised clinical studies, it has been observed that high-fat (plant-based) and low-carbohydrate diets are very effective in reducing the diabetes risk and complications with increased insulin sensitivity and improved lipid profile (high HDL and low LDL and triglyceride). In terms of quality of fat, higher intake of poly-unsaturated fatty acids (PUFA) and mono-unsaturated fatty acids (MUFA) were positively correlated to better insulin sensitivity as compared to the intake of high saturated fatty acids. Obese subjects with diabetes or insulin resistance display an altered fat and carbohydrate metabolism by high serum free fatty acid, insulin-resistant adipose tissue that limits the fat storage in them and higher accumulation of triglycerides in muscles that renders them insensitive towards insulin. Higher triglyceride leads to an increase in its degradation products such as diacylglycerols and ceramides that, if accumulated in β-cells, can leads to their failure and apoptosis (due to lipotoxicity). Such damage of β-cells leads to obvious insulin shortage and a resulting persistent hyperglycaemic state (glucolipotoxicity). It was also observed from various observational studies that consumption of coffee (three to four cups a day), tea (almost four cups a day), nuts and low-fat milk and dairy products have an inverse relation to the incidence of diabetes. As stated in previous chapters, diabetes and inflammation are very positively correlated and diabetes is often considered as an inflammatory metabolic disorder. It has been reported that diets rich in unsaturated fatty acids, arginine, magnesium and fibres reduce inflammation significantly and lower the incidence of diabetes [8]. A pictorial representation of the possible relationship between dietary pattern and diabetes is shown in Figure 8.1.

In another study on Indian participants reported more than a decade ago, it was found that lifestyle modifications such as brisk walking for at least 30 minutes per day, doing household activities and other physical exercise were very beneficial in resisting the development of diabetes in the people who were screened initially for impaired glucose tolerance (IGT). The addition of metformin did not result in any significant benefit [9]. In a recent study conducted on overweight or obese Mongolian population, it was observed that the mean body weight reduced significantly over a 6-month study period, while the HbA1c values of these subjects (initially in the diabetic range) reduced to the non-diabetic or pre-diabetic range after changing their dietary and physical work pattern [10].

At the molecular level, it has been experimentally verified too that restoration of damaged β-cells and their regeneration could be significantly achieved by changing the dietary pattern. In a recent study by Brereton et al., it was shown that the damage done to the β-cells is primarily due to the persistent hyperglycaemic state and later it becomes the other way around and acquires a cyclic process. Upon hyperglycaemia for 4 weeks, the insulin mRNA and protein reduced drastically, while that of glucagon increased significantly. Another important change observed was that many β-cells started

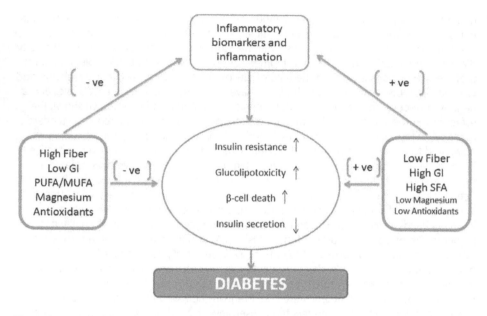

Figure 8.1 A possible relationship between dietary pattern and diabetes.

expressing glucagon on persistent hyperglycaemia. But the major point of this study was the fact that these molecular and structural changes (if any) were reversible once normoglycaemia is achieved [11]. In another very recent study on mouse models, it was observed that the fasting-mimicking diet (FMD; low-protein, low-carbohydrate, high-fat diet) led to β-cells' regeneration and production of insulin in diabetes mouse models. The researchers concluded that the FMD model led to an expression of the Ngn3 gene with greater insulin expression and secretion that is the basic characteristic of β-cells and that the FMD cycle could reverse the β-cell failure [12]. In a recent position statement published by the Academy of Nutrition and Dietetics, United States, it is suggested that medical nutrition therapy (MNT) can be highly beneficial in halting the progress of diabetes in pre-diabetes individuals and controlling diabetes in T2DM patients. It actually compiled the results of various clinical trials and suggested that in pre-diabetes subjects, at least 3 months of MNT reduced fasting glucose by 2 mg/dL to 9 mg/dL, body weight between 2.6 kg to 7.1 kg, and decreased waist circumference by between 3.8–5.9 cm. In the case of already established T2DM, the correct MNT resulted in a decrease of HbA1c by 0.3% to 2% after 3 months of nutrition therapy and the improvement was even more marked if the MNT continues. Several studies also reported a decrease in diabetes medicine (number, dosage or both) in subjects who took MNT sincerely [13].

Metabolic Effects of Exercise

In a recent position statement released by American Diabetes Education, it was well mentioned that aerobic exercise (such as walking, running, swimming, jogging) increases insulin sensitivity, mitochondrial density in the cells, immune function and cardiac output. Moderate to high amount of aerobic exercise is associated with significantly lower cardiovascular disease and related mortality and overall mortality risks in both T1DM and T2DM patients. It was reported that in T1DM patients, moderate aerobic exercise improved the endothelial functions, decreased the insulin resistance significantly and also improved the blood lipid levels. In T2DM patients, aerobic activities improved the HbA1c value, decreased blood pressure (if present), triglycerides and improved the insulin resistance. Apart from aerobic activities, resistance training such as weight lifting can also have beneficial effects on diabetes patients in terms of improvement of muscle mass (if there is a loss in muscle mass), improvement of bone mineral density, muscle strength, improved glycaemic control (in T2DM candidates), decrease in lipid profile, improvement of cardiac health and overall relieving mental state. It was stated that if aerobic and resistance exercise are to be done together one after the other, it is better to start with the resistance activity followed by aerobic exercise rather than the opposite, as the latter regimen can increase the risk of hypoglycaemia. Although as per the ADA, the effectiveness of alternative exercise regimens such as yoga and Tai chi is not well established, yoga can improve glycaemic control and lipid profile in T2DM patients. Prolonged sitting is highly discouraged in all, especially in diabetes patients. A brief 5-minute bout of standing or walking around after every 30 minutes of sitting is generally recommended to give glycaemic control in such individuals with desk jobs [14]. Aerobic, resistance or combined exercise have very beneficial effects on fat and glucose utilisation. There is a large mobility of stored and circulating excess fat towards the muscles for utilising them during the time of such exercises. There is an increased fat oxidation and utilisation during an exercise regimen. Lipolysis of adipose stored triglycerides tissue is seen to be greatly stimulated by an increase in the catecholamines concentration and action induced by exercise. Thus, exercise can have a beneficial effect on diabetes patients who are obese. On the glucose utilisation front, the rate of glucose uptake by skeletal muscles increases by many times during exercise. This is primarily attributed to an increased blood flow in the skeletal muscle cells and an increase in the GLUT-4 expression, translocation and activity. Interestingly, it is also stated that the exercise-induced increased GLUT-4 that pool in the skeletal muscle cells are distinct from those that are insulin-induced. Thus, there seems to be a direct glucose utilisation benefit from exercise. In terms of glycolysis, it has been stated that exercise increases the expression and activity of the hexokinase enzyme that phosphorylates glucose into glucose-6-phosphate, which is the first step of glycolysis. It has been said, though in animal studies, that increased expression of hexokinase led to an increased translocation of GLUT-4 and increased glucose utilisation. It was supported by the fact that overexpression and translocation of GLUT-4 alone did not result in sufficient glucose uptake without hexokinase expression. Since the GLUT-4 effect of exercise is distinct from the insulin-mediated GLUT-4 effect, it is seen that the effect of exercise in lowering blood glucose is significant even in T2DM patients who are insulin resistant. Apart from this short-term exercise-induced glucose uptake and utilisation, continuous aerobic or resistance exercise can improve the insulin-resistant state in T2DM patients by increasing the expression of various proteins involved in insulin-dependent glucose metabolism [15]. In a random controlled trial (RAED2 trial) on 38 T2DM patients by Bacchi et al. [16], it was found that although HbA1c improvement was almost the same in both the aerobic and resistance exercise groups, insulin sensitivity increased by almost 30% in the aerobic group, while there was a 15% increase in the resistance exercise group but no significant improvement in the β-cell function. There was a significant reduction in abdominal visceral fat in both groups. Another interesting finding states that genetic predisposition greatly influences the effect of exercise on people. It is shown that a single nucleotide polymorphism or SNP (rs540467) in the enzyme NADH dehydrogenase 1β sub-complex subunit 6 (*NDUFB6* gene) of mitochondrial complex 1 greatly impacts the ATP utilisation in an exercise regimen. T2DM patients (with non-responder allele rs540467 G/A) displayed only around a 33% rise in ATP synthase flux, while the non-T2DM patients with a responder allele (rs540467 G/G) showed around a 74% ATP synthase flux. In terms of percentage of subjects studied, almost 25% showed increased ATP synthase flux in the non-responder group, while almost 86% in the responder group displayed an increase in ATP synthase flux [17].

Another important, yet controversial, protein is irisin, which has been shown to be related to physical exercise. Irisin initiated a lot of debate and experiments after its first published report in 2012 by Bostrom et al. [18]. PGC1α, which is a co-activator of PPARγ, also increased thermogenesis by modulating the uncoupling protein-1 (UCP-1) in brown adipose tissue (BAT). Upon exercise, PGC1α is said to exert many beneficial effects such as mitochondrial biogenesis, increased blood flow and oxidative metabolism in skeletal muscles. It is also said to be helpful in resisting muscular dystrophy. Among many muscle proteins being influenced by PGC1α, a membrane protein named FNDC5 (fibronectin type III domain-containing protein 5) is processed and cleaved to generate irisin. Bostrom also stated that the irisin expression and secretion increases following exercise. But this research was later found to have several discrepancies and the report was largely discarded by the scientific communities [19, 20]. As an adipokine, it was reported that irisin is secreted much more from subcutaneous fat as compared to visceral fat. Similar to the case of leptin, researchers have also observed an irisin resistance in obese animal models. In an interesting possible relation with glucose regulation, high irisin expression has been found in islets and serous acinar cells in the pancreas. Irisin is said to have a positive association with circulating insulin levels and HOMA of β-cell function (HOMA-β) in subjects with normal glucose tolerance, indicating that the protein irisin might have an important role in the regulation of β-cell function. But there were contradictory results in other studies too. Several human studies have revealed a positive correlation between the irisin level and body weight or BMI. It has been observed that obese people had higher circulating irisin than people of normal weight, who in turn had higher circulating irisin than patients of anorexia nervosa. Similarly, it was also found that obese women with polycystic ovarian syndrome (PCOS) had higher levels of circulating irisin as compared to women of normal weight. It was also seen that diet-induced weight loss resulted in a significant fall in irisin levels, while the level returned to normal upon weight gain. As seen in animal models, irisin resistance could be a possible mechanism in obesity that results in a positive correlation between the circulating irisin level, BMI and obesity. In the case of normal non-diabetic individuals, the irisin level was shown to be positively correlated with insulin resistance and fasting glucose, though the association was weak. But surprisingly, irisin blood levels were shown to be lower in people with pre-diabetes and T2DM (though contradictory results are also present). However, still there has been no consensus statement on the association between irisin and metabolic syndrome because the result has varied outcomes in different populations [21]. In a patient-based study comprising 151 subjects on the relation of irisin and various parameters such as metabolic syndrome (including insulin resistance), adiponectin and other cardiometabolic variables, the researchers observed that the baseline irisin level was significantly higher in the subjects suffering from metabolic syndrome. Irisin was found to be positively correlated with BMI and negatively correlated with the serum adiponectin. Subjects with metabolic syndrome had a significantly lower adiponectin level. Irisin was also positively associated with systolic and diastolic blood pressure, fasting blood glucose and plasma triglyceride and insulin resistance. Higher irisin was found to be negatively correlated with HDL. The researchers concluded that an increase in irisin might be related to an increased risk of metabolic syndrome and CVD, and that there could be an effect of irisin resistance in those subjects [22]. In a later meta-analysis, it was shown that irisin was positively correlated with insulin resistance. It was also reported that increased irisin was associated with an increase in pro-inflammatory markers such as TNF-α, IL-6 and CRP [23]. In another recent study conducted on Egyptian patients (150 T2DM and 150 control), it was observed that the irisin level was significantly lower in T2DM patients, while it was higher in obese, non-diabetic patients. But in both the cohorts, serum irisin was positively correlated with BMI. This result was consistent with the finding that since PGC1α expression was significantly downregulated in the skeletal muscles of T2DM patients, irisin, which is positively influenced by PGC1α, is found to be decreased in T2DM subjects [24]. In a recent study conducted in China on 362 T2DM and 100 control subjects on the relationship between irisin level and advanced glycation end-products (AGEs), it was found that irisin was significantly lower in T2DM patients as compared to the age- and gender-matched control subjects. Since diabetes increases the AGEs in the body, irisin was found to be negatively correlated to the AGEs measured through the skin autofluorescence method. Though, as an inference, it was said that lower irisin was independently associated with an increase in AGEs [25]. In a very recent patient study on the effect of three different diets on the irisin level in subjects suffering from metabolic syndrome, it was found that at the baseline (before the study started), all recruited subjects with metabolic syndrome had a significantly lower irisin level as compared to the control group of people not suffering from metabolic syndrome. The study group was provided with low glycaemic index diets, Mediterranean diets and low glycaemic index, Mediterranean diets. After 6 months of the trial, the group that was provided with low glycaemic index diets showed a significant rise in irisin, while the other two groups did show a rise, but the difference was not significant. The study also observed a positive correlation between the irisin level and intake of vegetable proteins and saturated fats, while there was a negative correlation with cheese and processed meat. Though this study was performed in an Italian population, there have been certain discrepancies in different population studies, as stated earlier [26]. In a recent meta-analysis on irisin-related articles published between 2012 and 2016, it was suggested based on a total of 19 selected important articles that there have been very inconsistent reports on the relationship between diabetes and irisin level. On the one hand, various studies suggest a negative correlation, while several other have reported no significant correlation [27]. A positive correlation between irisin and T2DM was observed in another recent patient study. As consistent with various other results, irisin was found to be positively correlated with BMI and HbA1c. E-selectin is an adhesion molecule that has been found to be elevated in hyperlipidaemic and inflammatory conditions. E-selectin is not normally expressed but its expression is increased from activated endothelium and is highly responsible for leukocyte adhesion to the endothelium, leading to endothelial dysfunction. Irisin level was found to positively affect the expression and release of soluble E-selectin. This effect was verified *in vitro* too, where irisin exposure to primary human umbilical vein endothelial cells (HUVEC) resulted in almost a 2.5 increase in the expression and release of soluble E-selectin protein [28]. Thus, a consistent inconsistency has been observed in various studies linking circulating irisin levels with various parameters of diabetes and cardiometabolic conditions. As per our understanding, more *in vitro* and large population-based research is needed before coming to any conclusive remarks about the exact role of irisin in humans.

Thus, owing to the facts presented above regarding dietary and lifestyle modifications, it is widely evident that the quality of diet, pattern of eating, physical exercise and a mix of these are crucial in normalising the diabetes parameters in people with IGT or newly diagnosed diabetes. These interventions are very encouraging in people with long-term diabetes who are on medications. The fact that dietary modifications have significant positive changes in the insulin-producing β-cells supports that fact that diabetes can be treated as a reversible condition (to a great extent) even without medicines or fewer medicines. Dietary management has also shown to have positive effects on individual markers and proteins in diabetes and related comorbidities. *But, as a piece of precautionary advice, these interventions should ALWAYS be discussed with the healthcare provider and the registered dietary nutritionist before initiating to avoid any unfavourable circumstances resulting from fasting, especially in people who are on sulphonylureas or insulin as sudden hypoglycaemia could be detrimental at times.*

Gut Microbiome and Diabetes: Old Companion with a New Angle

Starting from birth, the human gut becomes the habitat of numerous microbes. This normal flora is highly useful as it is essential to various biochemical cycles inside the body. The constituent and quantity of microbes have been reported to change based on our activities such as dietary pattern, exercise habits, residential conditions, etc. Among these, diet has been considered the most important factor as it has been extensively studied. The co-metabolism by gut microbiota is essential in various macromolecule syntheses and the digestion process. It has also been stated that the gut microbiome dysbiosis results in chronic low-grade inflammation [29]. The human gut is primarily inhabited by Bacteroidetes sp. (gram negative) and Firmicutes (gram positive), which constitute approximately 90% of the total gut microbiota. The remainder is inhabited by actinobacteria (gram positive), proteobacteria (gram negative), verrucomicrobia (gram negative), fusobacteria (gram negative) and cyanobacteria (gram negative). One of the major functions of colonic microbiota is the colonic fermentation of insoluble fibres and oligosaccharides. This fermentation produces important short-chain fatty acids (SCFAs) such as acetate, propionate and butyrate. These SCFAs have very important physiological roles in colon physiology such as stimulating cellular proliferation of colonic epithelium, inhibition of intestinal inflammation and oxidative stress in that region and regulating glucose homeostasis [29]. The crosstalk among the gut microbiota (and with human cells) has recently come to light with the advent of better genomic tools and metagenomics concepts. It is gradually becoming evident that the gut microbiome is highly responsible for various physiological and pathophysiological states by influencing immunity, metabolic parameters, cardiological health, inflammatory responses, neuropsychological states and even cancer. The focus on the gut microbiome is also evident from a report revealing that almost 12,900 papers were published between 2013 and 2017 related to the matter. The gut microbiota population is predominated by bacteria and phages [30]. Though the earlier focus was on the relationship of gut microbes and complex carbohydrate digestion, strong recent evidence suggests that they have a much wider function and the regulation of metabolic, inflammatory and immune health of the host. Alteration in gut microbiota due to disruption in nutrition pattern or other pathological reasons can result in acute or chronic metabolic disturbances, resulting in insulin resistance due to initiation of inflammatory processes. It was also indicated that healthy non-diabetic individuals have higher butyrate-producing gut bacteria such as

Akkermansia muciniphila, Eubacterium rectale, Roseburia intestinals and *Faecalibacterium prausnitzii*, while the population of diabetic patients indicated a significant reduction in these species and a growth in opportunistic pathogens such as *Bacteroides caccae, Clostridiales* spp. and *Escherichia coli*. Desulfovibrio, a sulphate-reducing bacteria, was commonly observed in type 2 diabetes patients [31]. The healthy gut microbiota has been shown to produce enzymes that digest soluble dietary fibres to produce short-chain fatty acids (SCFAs). These SCFAs are reported to contribute towards 5–10% of energy source in healthy people. Moreover, it is a well-known fact that a fibre-enriched diet improves insulin signalling and sensitivity, thereby improving the blood glucose level. These SCFAs also act as prominent ligands activating GPCR 41 (free fatty acid receptor 3) and GPCR43 (free fatty acid receptor 2). It has been reported that binding of SCFAs to GPCR41 in L-cells of the small intestine and glucose results in secretion of GLP-1 that improves insulin secretion. This ligand-receptor interaction also stimulates the release of peptide YY, which inhibits the intestinal motility, increasing the transit time leading to increased nutrition absorption [29]. These GPCRs have been shown to be expressed in cells such as adipose tissue, gut epithelium and various immune cells. It was specifically mentioned that GPCR43-deficient animals are obese even after consuming a non-obesogenic normal diet, while the animals overexpressing GPCR43 in adipocytes remain lean even after consuming a calorie-rich diet. It was further reported that GPCR43 activation results in secretion of GLP-1 in the gut, thereby improving the insulin action and maintaining normoglycaemia [31].

In connection with type 1 diabetes, it was found and reported that type 1 diabetic children had increased *Bacteroides* and significantly decreased *Bifidobacterium* in their intestines. One study in Finland also found that the presence of the bacteria *Bacteroides dorei* preceded the presence of autoantibodies for T1D in children between 4 to 26 months of age. In the DIABIMMUNE study in Finland, it was found that in T1D children, Lachnospiraceae and Veillonellaceae spp. decreased significantly, while there was a marked increase in *Streptococcus* spp., *Blautia* and *Ruminococcus* spp. [32]. In a very recent publication in *Nature*, Vatanen et al. mentioned that various studies in Finland, Germany, Italy, Mexico and Turkey have reported that the gut microbiome dysbiosis is a key factor that promotes type 1 diabetes. The patients have an increased population of Bacteroides and a decreased population of probiotics that help in producing SCFAs. The TEDDY trial by Vatanen et al. specifically mentioned that the gut of healthy children contained useful SCFA-producing bacteria, mostly of the genus *Bifidobacterium*, and the species might change based on geographical location. But T1D patients lack these beneficial bacteria [33]. In a recent meta-analysis by Jamshidi et al., it was mentioned that the dysbiosis to a healthy gut microbiome is largely witnessed in T1D patients and the altered microbiome consisted of bacteria such as *Bacteroides* spp., *Streptococcus* spp., *Clostridium* spp., *Staphylococcus* spp. and *Blautia* spp. [34]. A recent report from Siljander et al. mentioned the fact that the dysbiosis in the gut microbiome occurs long before any sign of islet autoimmunity. This alteration has a significant impact on the immune system that drives the host body towards autoimmunity. The dysbiosis leads to increased intestinal permeability which leads to increased exposure to self and non-self antigens to the local immune cells and lymph nodes. It was also stated strongly that regardless of geographical location, the patients developing T1D displayed two common things viz. an increased proinflammatory response in the gut and a relatively increased population of Bacteroides and decreased population of Firmicutes. It was also mentioned that the genetic pool in the stool samples indicated more fermentation-related genes (for producing SCFAs) in healthy children than in T1D-affected children. The authors also mentioned in detail that few viral infections and the viral population of the gut could also be a key deciding factor behind development and progression of T1D [35].

In a review by Upadhyaya and Banerjee in 2015, it was mentioned that treatment with the bacteria *Akkermansia muciniphila* improved the metabolic parameters such as adipose tissue inflammation and insulin resistance in type 2 diabetes. Administration of *A. muciniphila* improved gut motility and permeability, while also controlling gut inflammation [36]. Microbiome analysis also revealed that butyrate (anti-inflammatory actions) producing Clostridia is found to be significantly less in the faecal matter of T2D patients. Metabolomic analysis among T2D and healthy patients also revealed an increased concentration of branched-chain amino acids in patients with insulin resistance, which was correlated with the increased presence of *Prevotella copri* and *Bacteroides vulgatus* [37]. A recent microbiota analysis by Allin et al. also revealed that friendly *Clostridia* spp. decreased significantly, while there was a significant rise in *Ruminococcus* and *Streptococcus* spp., in pre-diabetes individuals. A significant decrease in *A. muciniphila* is also reported in this large microbiota analysis. The *Clostridium* population was reported to show a negative correlation with fasting blood glucose and inflammation [38]. In light of pharmacological interventions, it has been widely reported that metformin increases the probiotic population with an increased production of SCFAs, which aids glucose homeostasis. Metformin was specifically shown to increase the population of *A. muciniphila* and *Bifidobacterium* [39, 40]. To gain a deeper insight into the role of gut microbiota, T2D and role of metformin, readers can refer to the reviews by Sircana et al. [41] and Rodriguez et al. [42].

REFERENCES

1. American diabetes association classification and diagnosis of diabetes: Standards of medical care in diabetes-2018. *Diabetes Care* 2018;41(Suppl 1):S13–S27.
2. Diabetes Prevention Program Research Group. Reduction in the incidence of type 2 diabetes with lifestyle intervention or metformin. *N Engl J Med* 2002;346(6):393–403.
3. Ratner RE. An update on the diabetes prevention program. *Endocr Pract* 2006;12(Suppl 1):20–24.
4. Nathan DM, Connor EB, Crandall JP, Edelstein SL, Goldberg RB, Horton ES et al. Diabetes prevention program research group. Long-term effects of lifestyle intervention or metformin on diabetes development and microvascular complications: The DPP outcomes study. *Lancet Diabetes Endocrinol* 2015;3(11):866–875.
5. Nowlin SY, Hammer MJ, D'Eramo Melkus G. Diet, inflammation, and glycemic control in type 2 diabetes: An integrative review of the literature. *J Nutr Metab* 2012;2012:542698.
6. McNaughton SA, Mishra GD, Brunner EJ. Dietary patterns, insulin resistance, and incidence of type 2 diabetes in the Whitehall II study. *Diabetes Care* 2008;31(7):1343–1348.
7. Forouhi NG, Misra A, Mohan V, Taylor R, Yancy W. Dietary and nutritional approaches for prevention and management of type 2 diabetes. *BMJ* 2018;361:k2234.
8. Salas-Salvado J, Martinez-Gonzalez MA, Bullo M, Ros E. The role of diet in the prevention of type 2 diabetes. *Nutr Metab Cardiovas Dis* 2011;21(Suppl 2):B32–B48.

9. Ramachandran A, Snehalatha C, Mary S, Mukesh B, Bhaskar AD, Vijay V. The Indian Diabetes Prevention Programme shows that lifestyle modification and metformin prevent type 2 diabetes in Asian Indian subjects with impaired glucose tolerance (IDPP-1). *Diabetologia* 2006;49(2):289–297.

10. Sonomtseren S, Sankhuu Y, Warfel JD, Johannsen DL, Peterson CM, Vandanmagsar B. Lifestyle modification intervention improves glycemic control in Mongolian adults who are overweight or obese with newly diagnosed type 2 diabetes. *Obes Sci Pract* 2016;2(3):303–308.

11. Brereton MF, Iberl M, Shimomura K, Zhang Q, Adreaenssens AE, Proks P et al. Reversible changes in pancreatic islet structure and function produced by elevated blood glucose. *Nat Commun* 2014;5:4639.

12. Cheng CW, Villani V, Buono R, Wei M, Kumar S, Yilmaz OH et al. Fasting-mimicking diet promotes Ngn3-driven b-Cell regeneration to reverse diabetes. *Cell* 2017;168(5):775–788.

13. Briggs EK, Stanley K. Position of the Academy of Nutrition and Dietetics: The role of medical nutrition therapy and registered dietitian nutritionists in the prevention and treatment of prediabetes and type 2 diabetes. *J Acad Nutr Diet* 2018;118(2):343–353.

14. Colberg SR, Sigal RJ, Yardley JE, Riddell MC, Dunstan DW, Dempsey PC et al. Physical activity/exercise and diabetes: A position statement of the American Diabetes Association. *Diabetes Care* 2016;39(11):2065–2079.

15. Moghetti P, Bacchi E, Brangani C, Donà S, Negri C. Metabolic effects of exercise. *Front Horm Res* 2016;47:44–57.

16. Bacchi E, Negri C, Zanolin ME, Milanese C, Faccioli N, Trombetta M et al. Metabolic effects of aerobic training and resistance training in type 2 diabetic subjects: A randomized controlled trial (the RAED2 study). *Diabetes Care* 2012;35(4):676–682.

17. Stephens NA, Sparks LM. Resistance to the beneficial effects of exercise in type 2 diabetes: Are some individuals programmed to fail? *J Clin Endocrinol Metab* 2015;100(1):43–52.

18. Boström P, Wu J, Jedrychowski MP, Korde A, Ye L, Lo JC et al. A PGC1-α-dependent myokine that drives brown-fat-like development of white fat and thermogenesis. *Nature* 2012;481(7382):463–468.

19. Accessed at https://pubpeer.com/publications/D58CD92ADD3D6301612B0C587147F0.

20. Accessed at https://retractionwatch.com/2017/02/27/coauthors-past-misconduct-prompts-dept-chair-retract-diabetes-study/.

21. Perakakis N, Triantafyllou GA, Fernández-Real JM, Huh JY, Park KH, Seufert J et al. Physiology and role of irisin in glucose homeostasis. *Nat Rev Endocrinol* 2017;13(6):324–337.

22. Park KH, Zaichenko L, Brinkoetter M, Thakkar B, Sahin-Efe A, Joung KE et al. Circulating Irisin in relation to insulin resistance and the metabolic syndrome. *J Clin Endocrinol Metab* 2013;98(12):4899–4907.

23. Qiu S, Cai X, Yin H, Zugel M, Sun Z, Steinacker JM et al. Association between circulating irisin and insulin resistance in non-diabetic adults: A meta-analysis. *Metabolism* 2016;65(6):825–834.

24. Shoukry A, Shalaby SM, El-Arabi Bdeer S, Mahmoud AA, Mousa MM, Khalifa A. Circulating serum irisin levels in obesity and type 2 diabetes mellitus. *IUBMB Life* 2016;68(7):544–556.

25. Li Z, Wang G, Zhu YJ, Li CG, Tang YZ, Jiang ZH et al. The relationship between circulating irisin levels and tissues AGE accumulation in type 2 diabetes patients. *Biosci Rep* 2017;37(3):pii: BSR20170213.

26. Osella AR, Colaianni G, Correale M, Pesole PL, Bruno I, Buongiorno C et al. Irisin serum levels in metabolic syndrome patients treated with three different diets: A post-hoc analysis from a randomized controlled clinical trial. *Nutrients* 2018;10(7). pii:E844.
27. de Alancar JP, Luna FMP, Coelho MB, de Morais RMRB, de Lima Neto JA, da Silva Filho MS et al. Low irisin levels in patients with type 2 diabetes mellitus without current treatment: A systematic review. *Int Arch Med* 2017;10(171), https://doi.org/10.3823/2441
28. Rana KS, Pararasa C, Afzal I, Nagel DA, Hill EJ, Bailey CJ et al. Plasma irisin is elevated in type 2 diabetes and is associated with increased E-selectin levels. *Cardiovasc Diabetol* 2017;16(1):147.
29. Fernandes R, Viana SD, Nunes S, Reis F. Diabetic gut microbiota dysbiosis as an inflammaging and immunosenescence condition that fosters progression of retinopathy and nephropathy. *Biochim Biophys Acta Mol Basis Dis* 2019;1865(7):1876–1897.
30. Cani PD. Human gut microbiome: Hopes, threats and promises. *Gut* 2018;67(9):1716–1725.
31. Tilg H, Moschen AR. Microbiota and diabetes: An evolving relationship. *Gut* 2014;63(9):1513–1521.
32. Paun A, Yau C, Danska JS. The influence of the microbiome on type 1 diabetes. *J Immunol* 2017;198(2):590–595.
33. Vatanen T, Franzosa EA, Schwager R, Tripathi S, Arthur TD, Vehik K et al. The human gut microbiome in early-onset type 1 diabetes from the TEDDY study. *Nature* 2018;562(7728):589–594.
34. Jamshidi P, Hasanzadeh S, Tahvildari A, Farsi Y, Arbabi M, Mota JF et al. Is there any association between gut microbiota and type 1 diabetes? A systematic review. *Gut Pathog* 2019;11:49.
35. Siljander H, Honkanen J, Knip M. Microbiome and type 1 diabetes. *EBiomedicine* 2019;46:512–521.
36. Upadhyaya S, Banerjee G. Type 2 diabetes and gut microbiome: At the intersection of known and unknown. *Gut Microbes* 2015;6(2):85–92.
37. Aydin O, Nieuwdorp M, Gerdes V. The gut microbiome as a target for the treatment of type 2 diabetes. *Curr Diab Rep* 2018;18(8):55.
38. Allin KH, Tremaroli V, Caesar R, Jensen BAH, Damgaard MTF, Bahl MI et al. Aberrant intestinal microbiota in individuals with prediabetes. *Diabetologia* 2018;61(4):810–820.
39. Vallianou NG, Stratigou T, Tsagarakis S. Metformin and gut microbiota: Their interactions and their impact on diabetes. *Hormones (Athens)* 2019;18(2):141–144.
40. Wu H, Esteve E, Tremaroli V, Khan MT, Caesar R, Manneràs-Holm L et al. Metformin alters the gut microbiome of individuals with treatment-naive type 2 diabetes, contributing to the therapeutic effects of the drug. *Nat Med* 2017;23(7):850–858.
41. Sircana A, Framarin L, Leone N, Berrutti M, Castellino F, Parente R et al. Altered gut microbiota in type 2 diabetes: Just a coincidence? *Curr Diab Rep* 2018;18(10):98.
42. Rodriguez J, Hiel S, Delzenne NM. Metformin: Old friend, new ways of action-implication of the gut microbiome? *Curr Opin Clin Nutr Metab Care* 2018;21(4):294–301.

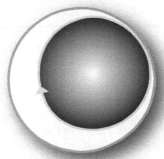

⑨ Future Prospects and Recommendations

In summary, we described in **Chapter 1** how diabetes has grown as a global metabolic epidemic from around 108 million patients in 1980 to almost 422 million in 2016. In a projected figure by the IDF, there could be around 642 million diabetes patients globally by 2040. Referring to specific nations, China and India are said to be the diabetic epicentres of the world. Undiagnosed diabetes, which may present itself at an advanced stage of the problem, remains one of the major global challenges. Among all forms of diabetes, type 2 diabetes affects the majority of the diabetes population, followed by type 1 diabetes mellitus. Other forms are monogenic diabetes, neonatal diabetes and gestational diabetes mellitus – all of which are described in the chapter. The chapter ends with a description of a special pathological condition known as diabetes insipidus which is not related to the hyperglycaemic condition, but received the name 'diabetes' due to excessive loss of water through urine which is very often also a cardinal sign of uncontrolled hyperglycaemia. In **Chapter 2**, diabetes is shown to be largely considered as an inflammatory metabolic disorder where inflammatory mediators play a vital role. Circulatory inflammatory markers such as TNF-α, IL-6, IL-1β, CRP and PAI-1 have been shown to be increased in diabetes. Immune cells that play a role in inflammation are also discussed in a comprehensive manner. The chapter also describes the interplay between various pro-inflammatory cytokines, chemokines and receptors in the development of insulin resistance and diabetes.

Chapter 3 deals with the concept of insulin resistance, which is often seen before diabetes develops. It shows the concept of how a large amount of free fatty acids is a foe of the human body, particularly to insulin signalling and glucose regulation. Excess accumulation of triacylglycerol also results in an increased concentration of ceramides which is also detrimental to islets. Various adipokines and cytokines play a major role in insulin resistance and glucose metabolism. The chapter also describes other aspects, including the effect of FFA on the protective adipokine adiponectin and the role of leptin in controlling eating behaviours. The chapter also deals with an interesting and burning topic of FGF-21 which has been shown to be greatly involved in glucose metabolism and insulin signalling. Another topic of interest is the role of high fructose in insulin resistance as various packaged food products now have a high amount of high-fructose corn syrup, which has been shown to be extremely 'bad' for health. Building on from that, **Chapter 4** describes the comorbidities arising due to persistent hyperglycaemia in diabetes. Unregulated diabetes, as described, can lead to a variety of problems and can technically damage almost all the organs and organ systems such as the cardiovascular system, kidneys, nervous system, eyes, lungs, reproductive systems, liver and even dental aspects, and can also lead to skin infections that are not healing and require tough interventions. The chapter provides a comprehensive collection of information regarding the brief molecular mechanisms behind those ailments.

Moving on from the diabetes-related comorbidities, **Chapter 5** deals with various biomarkers that are helpful in defining the diagnosis and prognosis of diabetes. **Chapter 6** describes various drug classes currently in use for diabetes treatment. The information consists of the basic molecular mechanism by which the drugs act and also various marketed drug forms along with their dosage regimen. At the end of this chapter, we have covered two important drug targets, the ligands of which are currently in various phases of pre-clinical and clinical trials. Moving on from the various drugs for diabetes, **Chapter 7** leads us to the diagnosis and treatment protocol as laid down by various authorities such as the ADA. The chapter describes the basic criteria of diagnosing T1DM, T2DM and GDM along with the treatment modality of T1DM and T2DM. But as is well known of diabetes, it is largely a disease deeply associated with eating habits and lifestyle patterns. **Chapter 8** deals with how lifestyle management and eating habit modifications can play a big role in controlling the onset of diabetes and also regulating the conditions once diabetes has been established. The chapter stresses how daily diet habits and physical exercise regimens have been proved to be highly efficacious in diabetes. It not only describes the quantity, but stresses that the quality of food is more important in controlling the condition of our bodies, especially if we are at risk of diabetes.

Index

Milton Keynes UK
Ingram Content Group UK Ltd.
UKHW040051071024
449327UK00019B/488